Staff Recruitment and Retention:

Study Results and Intervention Strategies

By

Sheryl A. Larson, Ph.D.

K. Charlie Lakin, Ph.D.

Robert H. Bruininks, Ph.D.

Research and Training Center on
Residential Services and Community Living
University of Minnesota

David Braddock, Ph.D.
Editor, Research Monographs and Books

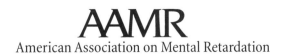

American Association on Mental Retardation

© 1998 by the American Association on Mental Retardation

Published by
American Association on Mental Retardation
444 North Capitol Street, NW, Suite 846
Washington, DC 20001-1512

Printed in the United States of America.

Library of Congress Cataloging-in-Publication Data
Larson, Sheryl A. (Sheryl Ann), 1963–
      Staff recruitment and retention: study results and intrevention strategies/
by Sheryl A. Larson, K. Charlie Lakin, Robert H. Bruininks ; David Braddock, editor.
                    p. cm. —
      Includes bibliographical references.
      ISBN 0-940898-56-X (pbk)
      1. Group homes for the developmentally disabled—United States—Personnel management. 2. Long-term care facililtes—United States—Personnel management. 3. Developmentally disabled—Institutional care—United States—Longitudinal studies. 4. Allied health personnel—United States—Longitudinal studies. 5. Paraprofessionals in social services—United States—Longitudinal studies. 6. Labor turnover—United States—Longitudinal studies.
      I. Lakin, K. Charlie. II. Bruininks, Robert H. III. Braddock, David L. IV. American Association on Mental Retardation. V. Title.
HV1570.5.U65L37   1998
362.1'6'0683—dc21   98-10508
                                         CIP

DEDICATION

This monograph is dedicated to the memory of Eunice Karlstrom, a great supporter and friend, who lived a long and rich life of service to her family, friends, and community; and Lynn Bachelder, a young, bright, and committed colleague and friend whose contributions to this field were cut far too short by her tragic death.

TABLE OF CONTENTS

LIST OF TABLES

ACKNOWLEDGMENTS

Inasmuch as this monograph is based on a dissertation completed by the first author, we begin by thanking and acknowledging the faculty members who participated in the project as the dissertation committee. Dr. Robert H. Bruininks, chair, Dr. Susan Rose, Dr. Richard Arvey, Dr. Jennifer York, Dr. Richard Weatherman, and Dr. James Brown provided advice, support, and encouragement in the development and completion of this project.

We thank Janet Bast, Stacey Tytler-Moore, Erin Simond, and Lynda Anderson who collected data, updated the project's data base, organized and recorded incoming surveys, typed and organized all of the quantitative responses to surveys, and who regularly contacted the homes in the study. These women contributed many long hours of dedicated work to make the details of this study come together. Dr. Amy Hewitt insisted that qualitative questions would be valuable, and she was correct. Thanks, Amy. Dr. Nahoon Kwak developed system files for this project and provided general statistical support, and Cheryl Morgan, Laura LaFrenz, Jennifer Sandlin, and Linda Schaffer provided timely secretarial support.

We thank the supervisors, direct support workers, advisors, colleagues and friends who helped with instrument development and pilot testing. We also acknowledge the agencies, supervisors, and direct support workers who participated in the study itself. They invested a great deal of time and effort in this study to learn more about how to improve support for direct support workers. Finally, we thank the Association of Residential Resources in Minnesota for endorsing this project.

The preparation of this manuscript was supported by cooperative agreements (#H133B0003-90 and H133D50037-96) between the National Institute on Disability and Rehabilitation Research (NIDRR) and the Research and Training Center on Residential Services and Community Living (RRTC), Institute on Community Integration, University of Minnesota; and through a cooperative agreement between NIDRR to the RRTC at the University of Minnesota (#H133B80048) through a subcontract from the Center on Human Policy at Syracuse University.

LIST OF ABBREVIATIONS

ANOVA	Analysis of Variance
AAUAP	American Association of University Affiliated Programs
ARRM	Association of Residential Resources in Minnesota
DAC	Developmental Achievement Center, also known as Day Training and Habilitation Programs
DD	Developmental Disabilities
DHS	Minnesota Department of Human Services
DSW	Direct Support Workers
FTE	Full-Time Equivalent
HCBS Waiver	Medicaid-funded Home and Community Based Services Waiver supports for persons with mental retardation
ICF-MR	Medicaid funded Intermediate Care Facilities for [persons with] Mental Retardation
LBDQ	Leader Behavior Description Questionnaire
MBA	Masters of Business Administration
MSQ	Minnesota Satisfaction Questionnaire
OCQ	Organizational Commitment Questionnaire
RJP	Realistic Job Preview
RTC	Regional Treatment Center
SILS	Semi-Independent Living Services
SLI	Staying or Leaving Index
SOCS	State Operated Community Services
Tech Prep	Technical job preparation initiatives

CHAPTER 1

EXECUTIVE SUMMARY: STUDY HIGHLIGHTS [1]

There are at least 305,000 paid full-time equivalent direct support positions in institutional and community residential settings for people with developmental disabilities in the United States. Nationally, in 1992 direct support workers earned an average wage of $5.97 per hour in private residential programs and $8.56 per hour in public residential settings (Braddock & Mitchell, 1992). National studies have found annual turnover rates for direct support workers in community residential settings ranging from 34% in small publicly operated homes to 70% for small privately operated homes, with most estimates of turnover rates in the 50% to 70% range (Braddock & Mitchell, 1992; George & Baumeister, 1981; Lakin & Bruininks, 1981; Larson & Lakin, 1992). With these turnover rates, at a national average cost per hire of $1,388 for nonexempt workers (JWT Specialized Communications, 1996), the cost of replacement staff could be as high as $212 to $296 million per year.

While staff turnover may produce both positive and negative outcomes, when turnover rates exceed 50% per year as they do in community residential settings, the problems outweigh the potential benefits. Confirmation that turnover rates are cause for concern for community residential settings comes from many sources. High turnover of direct support workers is a concern of consumers (Whiteman & Jaskulski, 1996), parents (Jaskulski & Whiteman, 1996; Larson & Lakin, 1991), community members (Governor's Planning Council on Developmental Disabilities, 1992), other direct support workers (Larson & Lakin, 1992), program administrators (Bruininks, et al., 1980; Larson, 1997), human services researchers (e.g., Braddock & Mitchell, 1992; Jacobson & Ackerman, 1989; Lakin & Bruininks, 1981; Zaharia & Baumeister, 1978), and policy makers (e.g., Department of Employee Relations, 1989).

Compounding the difficulties created by high turnover rates are increasing difficulties in recruiting replacement staff. Several reports have identified high vacancy rates and related recruitment problems for community residential settings (Coleman & Craig, 1981; Jaskulski & Metzler, 1990; Larson & Lakin, 1992; Larson, et al., in press; Legislative Budget and Finance Committee, 1989; Task Force on Human Resources Development, 1989). For example, in Minnesota an estimated 12% of direct support worker positions in residential service settings were vacant in August 1996 (Larson, 1997). Residential agency administrators reported that the average position

---

[1]**Note to readers:** This monograph describes a lengthy and complex research project. This executive summary is provided for those who want an overview of the study, its results, and its recommendations. A version of this executive summary was previously published as Larson, S.A. & Lakin, K.C. (1997). *A longitudinal study of turnover* *among newly hired residential direct support workers in small community homes serving people with developmental disabilities: Summary report.* Minneapolis: University of Minnesota, Center on Residential Services and Community Living, Institute on Community Integration (UAP). It is reprinted here with permission.

was vacant for 2.7 weeks before being filled, and that when they advertised vacancies only 7.3 applicants on average replied. Those administrators also reported that finding qualified staff members was their most difficult staffing challenge (71% reported it was a problem).

In recent years, finding direct support workers has become more difficult due to several demographic and labor market trends. The Bureau of Labor Statistics estimates that by the Year 2005, the number of home health aides will increase by 138% to 827,000, the number of human service workers will increase 136% to 445,000, the number of teachers' aides and assistants will increase 4% to 1.3 million, and the number of personal and home care aides will increase 130% to 293,000 (Leftwich, 1994). In addition, other service-related industries ranging from telemarketing to hospitality are growing rapidly. For every 10 newly created jobs in the United States, 8 are projected to be service oriented. However, the proportion of the U.S. population ages 18 to 44 (those who have historically been most likely to be direct support workers) is projected to drop from 42% to 37% between 1995 and 2005, and it will continue to drop even beyond 2005 (U.S. Bureau of the Census, 1996). Clearly recruitment and retention of community residential direct support workers is important both in research and in practice.

Methodology and Study Results

This study examines turnover among newly hired residential direct support workers through both facility-level and individual-employee-level analyses. In Study 1, facility-level analyses describe participating homes, examine turnover rates, and identify variables associated with facility-level turnover. In Study 2, individual-level analyses describe individual staff characteristics and identify individual and job-

related factors associated with turnover decisions. This summary reviews the methodology and results for each of these studies and then presents a combined discussion.

Study 1: Facility-Level Recruitment and Retention Issues

Methodology

One hundred twenty-eight of 188 agencies providing residential services to people with mental retardation in Minnesota in 1993 were screened for participation in this study. Of the 128 agencies screened, 94 (73%) were eligible for the study based on either being part of the Minnesota Longitudinal Study (a deinstitutionalization study also conducted by the University of Minnesota) or providing 24-hour residential services to people with developmental disabilities in at least one home with six or fewer residents. Administrators in 83 of the 94 eligible agencies (88%) agreed to participate in the study.

Homes were selected for the study using a two-phase process. In the first phase, supervisors of 116 homes were invited to participate, 108 based on being part of the Minnesota Longitudinal Study (see Hayden, et al., 1995) and eight based on being a State Operated Community Services (SOCS) home not in the Minnesota Longitudinal Study. Most of the homes selected based on their involvement in the Minnesota Longitudinal Study supported six or fewer people but a few were larger community facilities. In the second phase, 50 homes from randomly selected agencies not in the Minnesota Longitudinal Study that provided 24-hour supports to six or fewer people with developmental disabilities were recruited. One home was randomly selected from each participating agency. Supervisors in 143 of the 166 homes selected in Phase 1 and Phase 2 (86%) agreed to participate in the study. For this study 110 homes with six or fewer residents were included, 68 homes from Phase 1 and 42 homes from Phase 2.

Two facility surveys were completed by participating supervisors between December 1993 and December 1996. The first survey was administered when the home entered the study. The second survey was administered 12 months after the first survey was returned in homes still in the study. The facility surveys requested information about facility characteristics, staffing patterns, general staff characteristics, recruitment and retention challenges and characteristics of the people living in the home. A short form of the facility survey was used to gather basic information from supervisors unwilling or unable to complete the regular Time 1 or Time 2 facility survey. Supervisors in 143 homes competed the Time 1 survey and supervisors in 101 of 108 homes still in the study at Time 2 completed the Time 2 survey (94%). Among the 110 homes included in this analysis, Time 1 facility surveys were available for 110 homes, Time 2 facility surveys were available for 80 homes, and facility short surveys were available at Time 2 for 16 homes.

Results

Facility Characteristics. Of the 110 community residential settings included in this analysis, 43 (39%) were funded by the Medicaid Intermediate Care Facilities for [persons with] Mental Retardation (ICF-MR) program, and 67 (61%) were funded by the Medicaid Home and Community Based Waiver (HCBS) program. The average home opened in 1990 and served 4.7 people with developmental disabilities. The average cost per day per resident was $170 including room and board charges. Just over half of the homes (52%) were located in the Minneapolis/St. Paul metropolitan area while the rest were in out-state Minnesota.

Resident Characteristics. The people living in the participating homes could be characterized several ways. Most had severe or profound mental retardation (64%) and more than half (55%) had moved from a

state institution to this home directly. More than half had a specific intervention program to address challenging behavior, and one fourth (26%) had a formal diagnosis of mental illness in addition to mental retardation.

Direct Support Worker Wages and Benefits. Direct support workers earned on average $7.07 per hour starting wages, with the highest wage in each home averaging $9.27. Of the direct support workers in these homes, 43% were considered to be full time, 58% were eligible for medical or dental benefits, and 72% were eligible for paid leave time (holidays, vacations, paid leave).

Recruitment and Retention Outcomes. Supervisors reported that recruiting qualified workers was the most common staffing problem (reported by 57% of supervisors), followed by staff turnover (44%), and staff motivation (37%). Annual turnover rates averaged 46% for direct support workers and 27% for supervisors. Among the direct support workers who left the home during a 12-month period, 45% left within 6 months of hire, and another 23% left between 6 and 12 months after hire. Only 32% of those who left had more than 12 months' tenure in the home. Turnover and difficulties caused by turnover were measured twice in each home. While the average turnover rate did not change significantly from Year 1 to Year 2 (46% vs. 48%), the difficulty caused by turnover increased significantly during that period, $F(1, 94) = 4.19, p < .05$, from 2.8 to 2.6 (1 = very much, 4 = very little).

Factors Associated With Turnover. While the rate at which workers left the organization did not differ over time nor was it based on the type of facility, several other factors were associated with facility-level turnover rates. Variables with significant correlations with turnover at Time 1 included the population of the county in which the home was located ($r = .20, p < .05$), supervisor tenure in the home ($r = -.23, p < .05$), the proportion of direct support workers eligible for paid leave ($r = -.34, p < .01$), and the number of direct support workers promoted in the previous year ($r = .34, p < .01$). Turnover at Time 2 was significantly correlated with starting pay for direct support workers at Time 1 ($r = -.28$, $p < .01$), and supervisor tenure in the home at Time 1 ($r = -.24, p < .05$).

Two blocks of variables were tested to determine their contribution to explaining the variability in turnover rates. The first block consisted of context, facility, and resident characteristics that could affect turnover. The second block consisted of staffing patterns and strategies. A multiple regression analysis accounted for 34% of the variability (26% adjusted) in turnover rates at Time 1 using the following variables: unemployment rate, county population, average cost per resident, years home was open, ICF-MR status, resident case mix score, starting pay for direct support workers, whether live-in staff were used, the tenure of the supervisor in the home, and the percent of direct support workers eligible for paid leave, $F(10, 89) = 4.07, p < .001$. Unique contributions to explaining the variability in turnover rates at Time 1 were made by resident support needs, starting pay for direct support workers, supervisor tenure in the home, and the proportion of direct support workers eligible for paid leave.

Strategies to Address Staffing Challenges. Supervisors were asked to rank the importance of strategies they used to address staffing problems in their homes by identifying the five most important strategies they used. The most frequently identified strategies included encouraging team work among staff members (80% of all homes), managing fairly/treating staff members fairly (65%), communicating clear, understandable program objectives and agency philosophy (61%), establishing effective communication among staff members (45%), and using clear and understandable job roles and responsibilities (34%). Provid-

ing realistic job information was a priority strategy for only 25% of the supervisors.

An exploratory analysis was conducted to learn whether the strategies considered most important for addressing recruitment and retention challenges were associated with actual turnover rates in the homes at Time 1 and Time 2. Differences in turnover rates between homes in which the supervisors did or did not select each of the most popular strategies were tested using one-way analysis of variance. The use of direct observation to provide realistic information to recruits, and the provision of realistic information about the job to applicants as an important strategy were also tested. Of the top management practices identified by supervisors, only one was related to turnover. Supervisors who valued managing in a fair manner/treating workers fairly worked in homes with significantly lower turnover rates (40%) than supervisors who did not select fairness as a priority strategy (56%), $F(1, 94) = 6.16, p < .05$.

Interestingly, homes that used direct observation realistic job previews and homes that reported providing realistic information to recruits as an important technique had significantly higher turnover rates than the other homes (51% vs. 38% for homes using direct observations vs. homes that did not, $F(1, 94) = 3.84, p < .05$; and 61% vs. 40% for supervisors reporting realistic information as an important management strategy vs. supervisors who did not, $F(1, 108) = 7.54$, $p < .01$). It could be that supervisors in homes with higher turnover rates were more focused on the recruitment process because recent leavers said the job was not what they expected, or it could be that an emphasis on realistic job previews is associated with less focus on strategies associated with lower turnover rates.

Changes Impacting Outcomes. Supervisors were asked to describe any changes that had taken place in the agency or in their house that might have had an impact on staffing outcomes. Of the supervisors who identified specific changes, the most common changes reported were a new supervisor was introduced into the house (12% of all homes), the house had staff recruitment or retention problems such as a lack of qualified applicants (10% of homes), the support needs of residents changed (9%), and hiring or recruitment practices such as changing advertising strategies, using realistic job previews, or changing the person responsible for hiring new workers changed (8%). Other changes mentioned included improvements in staff training, improvements in management practices, changes in wages and benefits, and agency expansion.

Factors Related to Turnover (Supervisor Reports). Supervisors identified several factors that they felt influenced staffing outcomes. By far the most common factor was wages and benefits for workers (reported by 32% of all supervisors). Other important factors included flexible or fluctuating hours (14%), problems with team work or worker participation (14%), having mature, dependable workers (13%), providing good training (13%), providing consistent, effective communication for workers (12%), providing a fun or positive work environment (11%), and using innovating recruitment practices (11%). Other factors mentioned by more than one supervisor included the skills and characteristics of residents; fair treatment of employees; support and recognition for workers; supervisor training, qualifications, and style; clear expectations; and agency practices such as opportunities for advancement, location, and retention experience.

Supervisor Suggested Changes. Supervisors suggested ways the agency could make their job better. By far the most common response was to provide more or better training for supervisors (reported by 21% of all supervisors). Other common responses included improve agency communication (13%), use supportive management practices

(12%), and improve wages and benefits for workers and supervisors (9%). Other responses offered by more than one supervisor included help with time management, hire additional support staff, support supervisor decision making, reduce documentation requirements, address funding and budgeting issues, improve training for direct support workers, provide incentives for workers, and improve work space for supervisors

Study 2: Study of Newly Hired Direct Support Workers

Methodology

Five surveys were administered to up to three newly hired direct support workers in participating homes supporting six or fewer residents. The first survey was completed at hire and gathered information about personal characteristics, education and experience, job expectations, employment context information (such as quality of other job offers), and job characteristics. The second survey was completed 30 days after hire and gathered information about job characteristics (such as hours worked and salary), work-related characteristics (organizational commitment and job satisfaction), supervisor characteristics, employment context, training needs, and open-ended information about the job and how it could be improved. Two supplementary surveys were completed at the time of the second survey. One was the Leader Behavior Description Questionnaire, and the other was the Organizational Socialization Survey.

The third and fourth surveys gathered updated information about job characteristics (such as hours worked and salary), work-related characteristics (organizational commitment and job satisfaction), supervisor characteristics, employment context, training needs, and open-ended information about the job and how it could be improved. The third survey was administered after 6 months on the job and the fourth was administered after 12 months on the job. The final survey requested information from exiting employees about the person's leaving (e.g., was it voluntary, where did the person go), and about the good and bad aspects of the job. These surveys were administered in writing and were returned in sealed envelopes directly to the investigator. Supervisors completed an exit survey for direct support participants who left their position during the study.

A total of 174 of 333 (52%) direct support workers who were invited to participate in the study agreed. Of those, 124 who were new to the home and to the agency at hire were included in this analysis. All direct support worker participants worked regularly scheduled shifts (as opposed to on-call) at the home, and worked in homes supporting six or fewer residents.

Results

Direct Support Worker Characteristics.
Newly hired workers in this study were predominantly female (81%) and were an average of 28.8 years old at hire. Newly hired workers were overwhelmingly white (96%), unmarried (75%), with no financial dependents (76%). New hires had an average of 1.9 years of experience in developmental disabilities and had completed one and a half years of postsecondary education at hire. More than half (51%) of new hires had never worked in developmental disabilities prior to taking this job. Approximately one third (37%) of all new hires had taken a course on mental retardation, and 20% were currently enrolled in a postsecondary educational program.

Direct Support Worker Outcomes.
Of the 124 new hires in this study, 33% stayed in the same position for 12 months, 3% were promoted, 11% moved to another home in the agency, 38% left voluntarily, and 15% were terminated within 12 months of hire. An analysis of 58 workers who stayed 12 months and 47 workers who left revealed that stayers were significantly more likely than leavers to have heard about the job from inside sources (such as current or past staff members, family members, or friends) than outside sources (such as newspaper advertisements or employment agencies). Stayers were also significantly more likely to think they had a chance for a promotion than were leavers. Stayers had significantly lower intent to leave, higher organizational commitment, fewer unmet expectations, and higher extrinsic satisfaction than leavers. Overall 26% of the variability in staying or leaving was accounted for by organizational commitment, met expectations, alternative job opportunities, current salary, job satisfaction, supervisor structure, recruitment source, hours per week, months in field, age at hire, and intent to leave.

Reasons for Wanting to Leave. Workers identified several types of incidents that made them want to leave the home or quit the job. More than half of the workers (51%) said there were no incidents that made them want to leave, and another 23% did not respond to the question. Of those who did identify issues, the most common incidents were problems with co-workers such as staff talking behind each other's back (17%), inadequate pay, benefits, or incentives (16%), problems with supervisors (13%), and scheduling problems (13%).

Recommendations for Agencies. When newly hired direct support workers were asked what agencies could do to make their job better, the most common response was to increase or improve pay, benefits, or other incentives (37%). Another 33% of workers said no changes were needed because the employer or supervisor was doing a good job already. Other common suggestions included asking the supervisor to be more personable and attentive and to do a better job managing the home (17%), or to give the workers more, better, or different hours (17%).

Most Difficult Aspects of Direct Support Work. New workers also identified the hardest part of starting their job. Workers reported they had difficulty getting to know the people in the home and their behaviors and traits. This response was reported by 45% of all new hires. Another common response, reported by 43% of new hires, was that learning the routines and duties was difficult. A smaller, but still substantial, minority of new workers reported having difficulty getting to know and get along with other staff members (20%) and adjusting to the work schedule, particularly for those who worked overnight or early morning shifts (14%).

What Potential Direct Support Workers Should Know. The final question asked of new workers was what they would tell a best friend if the friend were thinking about applying for a job at this home. Workers mentioned several positive and challenging job features. Among the challenging job characteristics mentioned were behavioral or medical needs of residents (25% of workers), the need to work varying hours that included weekends and evenings (25%), and limited pay, benefits, and chances for advancement (20%). The most common positive characteristics mentioned included that the job was rewarding (19%), the work environment was good (19%), you have to be responsible and mature but can have fun (17%), and you will need lots of patience (17%). Study participants also advised potential workers to learn what duties are involved, be responsible and mature, be patient, and treat each person with dignity and respect.

Discussion

The direct support worker turnover rates in 110 community residential settings for people with developmental disabilities in Minnesota, averaging 46% to 48% over 2 years, were slightly lower than the reported national averages of between 50% to 70% annually (Larson, et al., 1994). They were much lower than the crude separation rate

of 67% reported for 25 randomly selected Minnesota community residences in 1992 (Braddock & Mitchell, 1992). But by the standards of virtually any industry, the rates are still very high, and they remain at levels that preclude adequately stable direct support for persons in small residential settings. In addition, many new hires were fired (15%). This termination rate remains identical to the one first reported for community residential settings nearly a generation ago (Lakin, 1981).

This study identified several factors that make a difference in recruitment and retention outcomes for community residential settings. One factor was the length a particular home has been in operation. For example, ICF-MR certified homes in this study, which opened much earlier than the HCBS Waiver funded homes, had significantly less turnover among direct support workers within the first 6 months of employment, had significantly higher average tenure, and hired significantly fewer new workers in a 1-year period. In addition, the average tenure of workers increased significantly overall between Time 1 and Time 2 in both types of settings. Both findings are consistent with previous studies, which identified length of operation as an important factor influencing turnover rates (e.g., Lakin, 1981).

It takes time for an agency to recruit and train a stable cadre of workers for a new home. Because the number of community residential settings nationally continues to expand rapidly (from 41,826 homes in 1992 to 78,365 homes in 1996; Prouty & Lakin, 1997), turnover challenges associated with opening new group homes and building a cadre of stable direct support workers are likely to continue as community supports continue to expand. Consequently, as new community residential options are developed, it continues to be important to identify and implement strategies to reduce turnover, especially during the first few years of operation of a new program. For individual organizations, pacing new developments may be important to avoid experiencing such "growing pains" at large numbers of an agency's sites. Spacing the development of new services appears particularly important in areas where unemployment is low, other job opportunities are high, and where wages and benefits in other service industries are highly competitive. Other strategies to reduce the effects of initially high turnover rates on agencies and the people they support suggested by this research include using some of the agency's established core of long-term employees from other sites (both supervisors and direct support workers) in new sites, increasing the proportion of positions offering full-time hours and benefits, and integrating a comprehensive program of recruitment and retention strategies into an agency's personnel practices. Elements of such comprehensive programs are identified in this monograph.

Resident characteristics appeared associated with direct support worker turnover when both were measured at the same time. Homes that served individuals with more challenging needs (in level of mental retardation, challenging behavior, mental health issues, or assistance with activities of daily living) tended to have higher turnover rates. As community homes are planned for people with more substantial support needs, particular attention should be paid to factors that minimize the turnover of workers. But personnel practices that adequately support direct support workers are needed irrespective of the needs of the people they support.

The tenure of supervisors in the home is a third factor related to turnover and retention of staff. Homes that had newer supervisors had higher turnover rates and lower average tenure than homes with more tenured supervisors. This is partially explained in that the maximum time a supervisor could have been in many homes was limited because many homes had opened within the last 5 years. However, supervisor tenure maintained its association with direct support worker turnover even after taking into consideration how long the home had been open. When supervisors were asked to identify factors that influenced direct support worker retention, the most commonly mentioned was supervisor turnover. In the facilities surveyed, the turnover rate for supervisors was 27% over a 12-month period.

The role of supervisors in affecting retention of direct support workers appeared very important in this study. Both staying and leaving direct support workers identified their supervisors as a key factor in leaving or wanting to leave the agency. Fair management practices were the second most common strategy identified by supervisors to address staffing problems. Direct support workers reported that having a competent supervisor was a very important expectation when they started their new jobs. Turnover rates were significantly lower in homes where the supervisors considered managing fairly to be one of their top five management practices. When supervisors were asked how the agency could help them do a better job, they requested training, improved communication, fair management practices by the agency, and support from the agency for staffing and recruitment issues. In developing interventions to address direct support worker recruitment and retention, the tenure, skills, and performance of supervisors were all important considerations.

It is, of course, impossible to overlook the importance of pay, benefits, paid leave, and promotional opportunities for the recruitment and retention of direct support workers. Starting pay accounted for a significant portion of the variability in turnover rates at the agency level. What's more, stayers were significantly more likely to report they thought they could get a promotion than leavers. Both direct support workers and their supervisors identified pay as a top factor influencing recruitment, retention, and plans to stay in the home. The availability of other jobs with better pay, working conditions or other conditions of employment was a significant predictor of whether direct support workers would stay or leave. Improving salaries, promotional opportunities and benefits for direct support workers is fundamental to increasing the stability of direct support workers.

The relationship between direct support workers and their colleagues emerged as an important issue in the qualitative data collection. Both supervisors and direct support workers reported that a sense of team work and positive relationships among direct support workers were important to overall staff retention. Among supervisors, it was tied for second among the factors viewed as influencing successful recruitment, retention, and training. Stayers identified problems with co-workers as the most common type of incident that made them want to leave. Leavers also reported that problems with co-workers had influenced their decision to stay or leave. Several workers complained that their co-workers gossiped about them, that competition among workers in different shifts was a problem, or that poor performing co-workers made their jobs more difficult.

Recommendations

Strategies to address recruitment and retention challenges in community residential settings include selection and recruitment changes, orientation and socialization practices, mentoring and training programs, and ongoing strategies such as enhancing the status of workers, training supervisors, and evaluating recruitment and retention outcomes.

Strategies for the Application Period

Selection Strategies

Several strategies can be implemented before a worker is hired to improve recruitment and retention experiences. Selection is the process used by organizations to improve matches between employee skills and organizational job requirements (Wanous, 1992). In this study, the rate of firings for new hires of 15% by the end of one year is an indication that improvements in selection practices could be helpful. Potential employees need to know specifically the criteria for disqualification for employment so that they do not invest their time applying for a job they will not be allowed to keep. Selection practices need to exclude workers who will be subsequently disqualified from employment because of their background check. Additional expense could be saved by recruiting new workers in anticipation of openings so that the background checks could be completed by the time the person is needed. This strategy has the additional benefit of reducing overtime costs incurred when positions are vacant for long periods.

Another selection strategy that may help recruits assess their own suitability for a job and employers assess the recruit is the structured interview. Structured interviews include the following key components: Each recruit answers the same set of interview questions; the questions address important behaviors that help distinguish excellent performers from poor performers; answers are evaluated using a predetermined scoring guide; and the questions ask recruits to describe experiences that relate to important job behaviors. One key challenge for supervisors is developing an effective team. A structured interview question might ask a recruit to describe a situation from his or her experience in which a co-worker did his or her job poorly or not at all. The interviewer would ask the recruit to describe the situation, what the recruit did, and what happened as a result. The answers would be scored based on descriptions of how well the recruit responded to such a situation.

Recruitment Sources

The pool of potential applicants for direct support work is not growing rapidly enough to provide an adequate supply of qualified workers. More effective recruitment efforts are clearly needed. Possible strategies include developing a volunteer program for students to introduce them to human services work; developing consortia of service providers in a geographic area to join recruitment efforts so that the field becomes more visible in the community; and developing specific recruitment materials such as brochures or videotapes that could be viewed by targeted pools of potential recruits in high school and college classes, job centers, employment agencies, and community centers (e.g., Hewitt & Larson, 1996); and developing public service announcements.

Recruitment incentives can also be helpful. Using incentive programs that pay bonuses when a new hire finishes a predetermined number of months on the job or a per recruit signing bonus for current workers can increase recruitment from inside sources. Besides increasing the number of recruits, incentive programs involving recruitment by current employees have the added benefit of recruiting people who were more likely to stay for at least 12 months (i.e., those recruited from "inside sources").

Recruitment Strategies: Realistic Job Previews

Realistic job previews (RJPs) are used to recruit people who will stay and do the job with personal satisfaction because they have a realistic impression of the job before they accept it. Components of realistic job previews include gathering information from new and long-term workers about the positive and negative characteristics of the job; summarizing information that recruits are unlikely to know or are likely to have unrealistic expectations about; developing a strategy to present the information to recruits before they decide whether to take the job; and implementing and evaluating the RJP. RJPs could include inviting prospective employees to a meal or recreational activity at the home; showing videotaped interviews with consumers, parents, and current staff members; showing a videotape of the typical household routines; delivering information about the job verbally to potential employees; or providing opportunities for potential employees to meet the people who live in the house and to observe the household routines. The goal is to provide a consistent set of nondistorted information about the job and the organization so that the recruit can make an informed decision about whether or not to take the job. Agencies who use a systematic realistic job previews for new hires consistently experience improved retention rates.

This study provided information that can be used to guide the development of RJPs. For example, direct support workers reported that what made them want to stay were the people in the home—both the residents and their co-workers—and the rewards of being needed. Some employees found the ability to tailor hours to their needs a positive aspect of the work. Others appreciated being a valued member of a team. Among the challenging aspects of the job for some workers were physically demanding resident behavior, low pay and inadequate benefits, problems with their co-workers and supervisor, and limited opportunities for advancement. Providing accurate information about these issues to new recruits early in the application process is an essential part of the recruitment process.

Strategies for Organizational Entry

Orientation Strategies

The most difficult job components for new workers in this study as they started their jobs were becoming acquainted with the residents, learning the routines, developing relationships with co-workers, remembering training information, and adjusting to the schedule. Many expressed concern about fulfilling the substantial responsibilities given to them. The experience of entering a new organization is stressful for all workers, but is made more so when responsibility is high and direct expert support and supervision is limited as is increasingly the case in small community-service settings. Agencies can help by communicating that the struggles facing the newcomer are typical and by providing specific suggestions about how to handle the stress they may experience. A successful orientation program will reduce the anxiety of new employees and make them feel a part of the organization; promote positive attitudes toward the job and the organization; establish open communication between the organization and the employee; communicate the expectations the organization has regarding performance and behavior; acquaint new employees with organizational background, goals, philosophies, management styles, structure, products, and services; and present information on organizational policies, procedures, compensation practices, and benefits (Holland & George, 1986). Providing planned opportunities for new workers to get to know other workers and the people they will be supporting before the first solo shift can be helpful in the orientation process. Pacing the information provided during orientation can also help to reduce the likelihood that a new worker will become overwhelmed with the information.

Initial Socialization

Deinstitutionalization has led to widespread decentralization of services and supports. Workers who previously would have had many co-workers at the same site now may be the only worker at the site at certain times or may have only one co-worker. However, this shift has produced new demands, challenges, and stressors for direct support workers. It is a particular challenge to develop strategies to support workers who are in scattered sites. People need to know how to get help and to feel confident that the help they need will be available. Providing such critical information and comforts is an important part of the initial socialization process. Some agencies enhance initial socialization efforts by introducing new workers to all of the homes in a geographic area so that there is always someone to call for advice or assistance.

The findings of this study also suggest that it is important during the initial socialization period to provide team building opportunities so that newcomers can feel integrated into the social environment of the home and agency. Considering that workers in some homes enjoyed their colleagues while others wanted to leave because of their co-workers, attention to team building and dealing with differences and disagreements among co-workers is important at the beginning of employment and on an ongoing basis.

Strategies for Organizational Socialization

Peer Mentoring

One of the most effective ways to accomplish the long-term socialization goals is to assign a mentor to new employees to help them through the first 3 to 12 months on the job and beyond. Mentoring programs can use peer mentors (workers in the same position as the new hire) or agency mentors (workers higher in the hierarchy than the new hire but not in the new hire's direct chain of command). Successful mentoring programs identify and match mentors carefully by selecting voluntary mentors based on fair, attainable, and known criteria; train both the mentors and the new employees about how mentoring programs work; train mentors on empathic listening, conflict resolution, providing feedback, leadership, and instructional techniques; and monitor, evaluate, and change the program as needed. Mentoring can reduce isolation of direct support workers and increase supports. It can also allow supervisors to delegate the tasks of answering routine questions about the job. Peer mentors benefit by developing a broader understanding of the work and of their co-workers.

Competency-Based Training

Training of new direct support workers is important because it is a direct regulatory mandate for most human services agencies (Larson, et al., 1994); it is considered a key element in achieving higher quality services (Alpha Group, 1990; Fiorelli, et al., 1982); it provides the opportunity to learn critical job functions, develop new skills, and cope with job roles (Camp, et al., 1986); and it develops attitudes and skills among employees that affect the quality of life for individuals with developmental disabilities (Jones, et al., 1981). A study of 1,736 new hires in different organizations suggested that workers who complete more weeks of training ($m = 4.5$ weeks of training for workers who stayed more than 7 months) had significantly lower turnover than workers in agencies with fewer weeks of training ($m = 1.9$ weeks of training for workers who voluntarily resigned) (Wanous, et al., 1979). Voluntary leavers also were less likely to receive informal job training (20% for leavers vs. 43% for stayers).

Ongoing Strategies

Enhancing the Status of and Opportunities Available to Direct Support Workers

Some efforts to enhance the status of and opportunities available to direct support workers can be made at the agency level through reorganization that flattens agency hierarchy, through restructured wage packages that offer at least prorated paid leave time for all workers, and through flexible paid leave time and benefits policies that allow workers to use those benefits as needed in their own particular circumstances. Other efforts require systemic change. New employment benefits may be needed. Some of these could be developed in conjunction with public agencies. These might include tuition credits at public colleges, universities, and technical schools. Alternatively, tax credits can be developed to allow retirees on Social Security to benefit from employment in supporting people

with disabilities. Even with these changes, however, public attitudes about the value of direct support workers as expressed in public policies about funding for residential services must change if large scale improvements are to be made.

Another way the status of direct support workers can be improved is through providing staff development and career advancement opportunities. In this study, stayers were significantly more likely to think promotional opportunities were available to them than were leavers. Providing employee bonuses for skill development, promoting workers from within, providing educational benefits, and developing career ladders are all important to improving the stability and quality of the direct support workforce.

Developing Links With Higher Education

The Kennedy Fellows Mentoring Program provides scholarships and career mentoring to direct support workers enrolled for at least six credits in two New York colleges (Hewitt, et al., 1996). This program encourages direct support workers to complete a 2-year degree, and helps them become eligible for promotions to positions with greater responsibility. Fifteen other states have federally funded Training Initiative Projects designed to identify, develop, and disseminate state-of-the-art training curricula; provide technical assistance and training to direct support workers, supervisors, agencies, consumers, and families, develop career ladder opportunities for direct support workers; complete training needs-assessments; and facilitate collaboration among key stakeholders regarding direct support issues (AAUAP, 1996). These projects reflect the growing national interest in and concern for developing, respecting, and supporting direct support workers. They also reflect examples of programs that can increase the visibility of careers in direct support work and can assist in recruiting new workers to the industry.

Staff Development for Supervisors

This study demonstrated an association between supervisor behavior and recruitment and retention outcomes. Homes with less tenured supervisors had significantly higher turnover rates. Addressing turnover among direct support workers may well begin with success in increasing stability among supervisors of the settings in which they work. Common practices such as rotating supervisors through settings may be detrimental to stability.

Staff development for supervisors is also important. Direct support workers identified having a good supervisor as an important issue, and reported that problems with supervision influenced their decisions to stay or leave. Supervisors also requested assistance. Training should be developed for supervisors on recruitment and retention strategies and leadership and supervision skills.

Ongoing Internal Evaluation of Efforts

It is not sufficient for an agency to have a general idea that it has a problem with recruitment or retention. Agencies need many different types of information to monitor recruitment and retention outcomes and to design effective intervention strategies. The components of a workplace assessment include developing an accurate job description; examining retention outcomes and recruitment practices; gathering specific information about positive and negative job features; describing any changes or special incentives that may have influenced recruitment or retention; and summarizing the information gathered. More detailed information about developing and using workplace assessments is available from the authors.

Conclusions

This society has made a clear commitment to the presence and participation of people with developmental disabilities in its communities, schools, and workplaces. That commitment is in jeopardy. Demographic shifts depleting the numbers of young adults, economic growth resulting in more available jobs, increasing wages, human service expansion, and other factors are making it increasingly difficult to maintain current levels of staff much less to expand the number of staff available to meet needs stemming from future growth. There is a crisis in the community that derives from what has been inadequate attention to the intractable connection between community living for people with disabilities and community supports provided by direct support workers.

The problems of recruiting and retaining direct support workers will continue to demand concerted and creative efforts by public officials, advocates, service providers, and others who care about the well-being of persons with developmental disabilities. Areas of particular focus include increased amounts and attractive options in compensation; more comprehensive and more effective recruitment initiatives; improved quality, recognition, and transferability of training; expanded career opportunities; more effective supervision; better matching of employees to work roles; and more effective team building. Success in these efforts is one of the most important components to assuring that community living is a real and viable option for all Americans with developmental disabilities.

We must not encourage the respect and dignity of one group of people (those with developmental disabilities) at the expense of another group of people (those paid to support them). Americans talk often of the importance of having good teachers for our children. We value those who would help children to become productive citizens of this nation. We must also respect those who help and support people with mental retardation and other developmental disabilities.

CHAPTER 2
WHY STUDY RECRUITMENT AND RETENTION: A RATIONALE

As primary providers of support, training, supervision, and personal assistance for persons with developmental disabilities in residential settings, direct support workers have considerable influence on the experiences, opportunities, and quality-of-life outcomes experienced by those individuals (Larson, et al., 1994). While the exact number of direct support workers is unknown, using staffing ratios from a report on ICFs-MR of various sizes in 1992 (Larson & Lakin, 1995), the staffing ratios in non-ICF-MR residential settings from the 1987 National Medical Expenditures Survey (Lakin, et al., 1989), and a report of the number of people with mental retardation living in staffed homes of various sizes in 1996 (Prouty & Lakin, 1997), it can be estimated that there are at least 305,000 paid full-time equivalent direct support positions in institutional and community residential settings for people with developmental disabilities. Unfortunately, direct support workers are often poorly paid (Braddock & Mitchell, 1992; Knight & Hayden, 1989), inadequately trained (Minnesota State Technical College Task Force, 1993), and likely to leave their positions quickly. Nationally, in 1992 direct support workers earned an average wage of $5.97 per hour in private residential programs and $8.56 per hour in public residential settings (Braddock & Mitchell, 1992). National studies have found annual turnover rates for direct support workers in community residential settings ranging from 34% in small publicly operated homes to 70% for small privately operated homes, with most estimates of turnover rates in the 50% to 70% range (Braddock & Mitchell, 1992; George & Baumeister, 1981; Lakin & Bruininks, 1981; Larson & Lakin, 1992).

Staff turnover has the potential to create both positive and negative outcomes for agencies and staff. On the positive side, turnover may displace poor performers, infuse new people with new ideas into the organization, increase the receptivity of the workforce to change, produce increased innovation, reduce conflict among co-workers, reduce personnel costs, and create promotion opportunities (Bluedorn, 1982; Dalton & Todor, 1982; Mobley, 1982; Muchinsky & Morrow, 1980; Price, 1989; Williams & Livingstone, 1994). On the negative side, turnover may cause co-workers to reevaluate their commitment to the company; increase administrative costs for selection, recruitment, training, and development; increase operational disruption; and disrupt communication and socialization patterns (Bluedorn, 1982; Bycio, et al., 1990; Muchinsky & Morrow, 1980; Mueller & Price, 1989; Staw, 1980; Steers & Mowday, 1981). Among direct support workers in residential settings, researchers have theorized that turnover may lead to discontinuity of treatment and care, chronic low productivity and staff shortages, increases in the relative size of the administrative staff, and increases in hiring and training costs (Lakin, 1988).

Turnover is not just a cause for concern; it is a costly problem in the developmental disabilities industry. A 1996 nationwide study calculated the costs to hire a nonexempt worker (an hourly employee in any industry) of at least $1,388 (JWT Specialized Communications, 1996). Zaharia and Baumeister (1978) estimated the cost of replacing a direct support worker in an institution to be $1,563 in 1976 or $4,304 in 1996 dollars. Given at least 305,000 full-time equivalent direct support workers in the United States and a turnover rate of 50%, the cost of hiring replacement staff could range anywhere from $212 to $656 million annually. A recent study of 144 randomly selected residential, vocational, in-home support, and mental health agencies in Minnesota (of 488 eligible agencies) provided more recent estimates of recruitment difficulties and costs. Annual advertising costs for all 488 agencies were estimated at $60 per position in 1996 with overtime costs adding an estimated $145 per position annually (Larson, et al., 1997). Minnesota community residential service agencies employ an estimated 32,503 direct support workers. With turnover rates averaging almost 50% annually, 15,252 existing direct support positions have to be filled each year in addition to the more than 3,000 newly created positions.

While staff turnover may produce both positive and negative outcomes, when turnover rates exceed 50% per year as they do in community residential settings, the problems outweigh the potential benefits. Confirmation that turnover rates are cause for concern for community residential settings comes from many sources. High turnover of direct support workers is a concern of consumers (Whiteman & Jaskulski, 1996), parents (Jaskulski & Whiteman, 1996; Larson & Lakin, 1991), community members (Governor's Planning Council on Developmental Disabilities, 1992), other direct support workers (Larson & Lakin, 1992), program administrators (Bruininks, et al., 1980; Larson, 1997), human services researchers (e.g., Braddock & Mitchell, 1992; Jacobson & Ackerman, 1989; Lakin & Bruininks, 1981; Zaharia & Baumeister, 1978), and policy makers (e.g., Department of Employee Relations, 1989). Compounding the difficulties created by high turnover rates are increasing difficulties in recruiting replacement staff. Several reports have identified high vacancy rates and related recruitment problems for community

residential settings (Coleman & Craig, 1981; Jaskulski & Metzler, 1990; Larson & Lakin, 1992; Larson, 1997; Legislative Budget and Finance Committee, 1989; Task Force on Human Resources Development, 1989). For example, in Minnesota an estimated 8% of direct support worker positions in residential service settings were vacant in August 1996 (Larson, et al., in press). Residential agency administrators reported that the average position was vacant for 2.6 weeks before being filled, and that when they advertised vacancies, only 6.3 applicants on average replied. Those administrators also reported that finding qualified staff members was their most difficult staffing challenge (75% reported it was a problem).

In recent years finding direct support workers has become more difficult due to several demographic and labor market trends. The difficulty in finding workers comes first from the rapid increase in the demand for direct support workers. The Bureau of Labor Statistics estimates that by the year 2005, the number of home health aides will increase by 138% to 827,000; the number of human service workers will increase 136% to 445,000; the number of teachers' aides and assistants will increase 4% to 1.3 million; and the number of personal and home care aides will increase 130% to 293,000 (Leftwich, 1994). In addition, other service-related industries ranging from telemarketing to hospitality are growing rapidly. For every 10 newly created jobs in the United States, 8 are projected to be service oriented.

The second source of difficulty comes from the relative decline in the available workforce. A review of 10 studies describing the characteristics of direct support workers noted that the vast majority of direct support workers are women under the age of 40 (Larson, et al., 1994). The proportion of the U.S. population ages 18 to 44 (those who have historically been most likely to be direct support workers) is projected to drop from

42% to 37% between 1995 and 2005 (U.S. Bureau of the Census, 1996). Clearly recruitment and retention of community residential direct support workers is important both in research and in practice.

Statement of the Problem

Research has identified many factors contributing to turnover of employees (see Chapter 3 for a detailed description of this literature). Well-tested turnover models, and several meta-analytical studies have identified variables consistently related to turnover. The major challenge now is to apply the knowledge from the literature to turnover among staff in agencies serving people with developmental disabilities, and to focus on periods of employment associated with the highest rates of turnover. Specifically, it is important to improve understanding of the variables associated with turnover among newly hired direct support workers in small community-residential settings serving people with developmental disabilities in the initial stages of employment when turnover is highest (i.e., during the first 12 months of employment).

The study described in this monograph applies and extends findings from previous research to turnover among newly hired direct support workers in small community-residential settings. It extends previous research in several respects. First, it examines turnover in small community settings, the largest and the only growing sector of the residential services system. Second, it focuses on turnover among newly hired workers, attending to those direct support workers with the highest rates of turnover, and examines organizational socialization during the crucial first 6 months on the job. The focus on newly hired workers promotes identification of interventions to reduce turnover of new hires that can be implemented in the recruitment, hiring, or orientation process. A focus on newly hired direct support workers allows separation of the effects of age from the effects of length of service on turnover by holding length of service constant. Finally, this study explores interventions suggested to improve recruitment and retention practices and gathers and reports supervisor and direct support worker suggestions and recommendations in this regard.

Additional refinements derive from the research design and methodology. First, this study uses both the individual employees and facilities as units of analysis. The facility-level analysis allows comparison of variability in turnover associated with facility variables with the variability in turnover associated with individual variables. The individual employee analyses refine the developmental disabilities' turnover literature by including variables from the rapidly growing personnel psychology literature that have not been systematically integrated into personnel studies in developmental disabilities. Second, this study uses a longitudinal approach in examining turnover, thereby incorporating actual leaving as the dependent variable rather than tenure or intent to leave and facilitating stronger inferences about causality. Third, the study identifies voluntary versus involuntary leaving, allowing a focus on individually motivated turnover. Finally, this study measures turnover over a 12-month period to span the interval in which 50% of new hires would predictably leave. This provides for the strongest possible statistical test of the variables included.

Beyond these methodological refinements, this research also identifies and, to a limited extent, evaluates specific intervention strategies to improve recruitment and retention. It examines the type, source, and extent of information available to new hires when they accept a position. It compares inside recruitment sources (such as getting information from a friend who works in the house or agency) with outside recruitment sources (such as newspaper advertisements), with regard to job tenure. It compares agencies using specific recruitment and retention strategies with regard to differences in turnover rates. It also reports recommendations of both supervisors and new workers about information that might be useful in designing improved recruitment and socialization practices.

Research Questions

This study examines turnover among newly hired residential direct support workers through both facility-level and individual-employee-level analyses. Facility-level analyses describe participating homes, examine turnover rates, and identify variables associated with facility-level turnover. Individual-level analyses describe individual staff characteristics and identify individual and job-related factors associated with turnover decisions. Specific research questions are as follows:

Facility-Level Analyses

1. What are the contextual, agency, facility, and resident characteristics of small homes supporting people with developmental disabilities?
2. What are the characteristics and roles of supervisors in small homes supporting people with developmental disabilities?
3. What are the staff characteristics, staffing patterns, and typical roles for direct support workers in small homes supporting people with developmental disabilities?
4. What are the conditions of employment (probation, promotion, wages, and benefits) for direct support workers in small homes supporting people with developmental disabilities?
5. How do recruitment and retention outcomes for homes funded under ICF-MR rules differ from those funded under Medicaid HCBS Waiver rules? How do these outcomes change over time?

6. What proportion of variability in annual turnover rates for small residential facilities is accounted for by facility characteristics?
7. What strategies are used to address recruitment and retention challenges in small Minnesota homes supporting people with developmental disabilities?
8. Does turnover vary depending on the use of certain intervention strategies identified by supervisors?
9. What factors and changes do supervisors report as influencing recruitment and retention outcomes?
10. What strategies do supervisors and agencies use and what strategies do they recommend using to address recruitment and retention challenges?
11. What assistance do supervisors need to do their jobs better?

Individual-Level Analyses

1. What are the personal characteristics, recruitment experiences, employment context, job expectations, job attitudes, and socialization experiences of newly hired direct support workers, and how do they differ for those who stay/leave in the first 12 months after hire?
2. What are the survival rates for newly hired direct support workers in community residential settings?
3. What proportion of variability in turnover among newly hired direct support workers is accounted for by personal characteristics, work-related characteristics, context variables and job characteristics?
4. Why do direct support workers leave a position? What could the agency do to make the job better?
5. What are the greatest training needs of newly hired residential direct support workers?
6. What information is important to tell to new applicants? What are the most difficult parts of the job for a newcomer?

CHAPTER 3
LITERATURE REVIEW

A vast amount of information about recruitment and retention challenges has been published during the last 100 years. For this project more than 1,000 published and unpublished monographs, studies, literature reviews, and other resources developed since 1963 were consulted. This literature review presents highlights of those studies. In the first section we review the literature that has been developed specifically by and for the developmental disabilities industry around workforce development issues. In the second section, we review the literature more broadly to point out the highlights of findings on workforce issues from other industries. This chapter also reviews information on the potential causes of turnover and on potential solutions for the workforce challenges faced by many industries including developmental disabilities.

Studies of Workforce Turnover in the Developmental Disabilities Literature

Administrators and researchers of developmental disabilities services have been investigating and expressing concern about turnover in residential settings since at least 1912 (Kirkbride, 1912). This research initially focused on institutional settings but now also examines community residential settings. Several detailed reviews of this research have been published (Baumeister & Zaharia, 1987; Braddock & Mitchell, 1992; Lakin, 1988; Lakin & Bruininks, 1981; Lakin & Larson, 1992; Larson, et al., 1994).

One literature review examining variables in turnover research noted that 73 different variables had been included in eight studies in institutional or community residential settings, but that only 14 variables

had been included in more than one investigation (Lakin & Larson, 1992). Of these, for 10 variables the direction of statistically significant findings were consistent. Higher turnover was associated with lower staff pay, more residents per staff member, urban location, homes open for a shorter time, low community unemployment rates, younger staff members, a staff with less tenure, supporting people with fewer adaptive behavior skills, supporting people with higher IQ scores, and supporting people in smaller homes.

Correlational data are useful in identifying variables that may have important associations with turnover, but they do not allow assessment of how, in what combination, and to what extent a set of variables can actually predict turnover. Tables 1 through 4 summarize all of the available studies that used multiple regression analysis to examine variables associated with turnover within developmental disabilities research. Table 1 shows three statewide studies that identified variables accounting for a statistically significant 16% to 34% of the variability in facility turnover rates. None of the studies at the facility level explained more than 34% of the variability in turnover. Of the variables in these studies, only the skill level of residents appeared as a predictor in more than one study. These studies were limited primarily in geographic scope (one state) and sample sizes (fewer than 50 facilities were studied in two of the three studies). The third study included both residential and vocational settings in the analysis.

Table 2 shows the findings of four recent single state studies using multiple regression to examine factors related to intended or actual leaving by individual employees. Pay or satisfaction with pay was significantly related to turnover in two studies, support from supervisors or co-workers was related to turnover in three studies, and job satisfaction was related to turnover in two studies. In these studies measurements of turnover or intent to leave at the individual level predicted a higher proportion of variability than the studies that measured turnover at the facility level. They also included variables, such as job satisfaction, support, and commitment, that were not routinely measured in previous studies. Only Bachelder and Braddock (1994) and Razza (1993), however, measured actual staying or leaving. The other studies used a proxy measure of turnover (e.g., intent to leave). As with the studies in Table 1, these studies were limited to a single state, and with one exception (Bachelder & Braddock, 1994) were limited to direct support workers in nine or fewer agencies.

Three studies have investigated turnover among large national samples of facilities (see Table 3). In all three studies, the number of direct support workers or the ratio of workers to residents was related to turnover. In two studies, starting salary was related to turnover. However, none of these studies using a facility level of analysis could account for more than 10% of the variability in turnover with the variables examined.

Table 4 summarizes findings from two national studies that examined turnover from an individual level of analysis. Lakin and Bruininks (1981) used a prospective approach to identify variables predicting whether individual direct support workers would stay or leave during a 1-year period. Larson and Lakin (1992) used a cross-sectional approach in which intended length of stay for current direct support workers was the dependent variable. Both studies found length of employment and previous special training to be predictors of staying or leaving. Tables 3 and 4 report data from the same investigations, but the proportion of

Table 1. Single State Multiple Regression Studies of Facility-Level Turnover

Authors	Subjects	R^2	Variables Contributing to Prediction of Variance
Department of of Employee Relations, 1989	252 facilities (including group homes, day programs, semi-independent living services, and rehabilitation facilities)[a]	16%	Average hourly pay ICF-MR certification status Region of the state
George & Baumeister, 1981	12 small agencies (Mean = 6.41 residents) 26 large agencies (Mean = 12.64 residents)	34%	Length of unit operation Age of residents Number of residents with severe behavior problems Community skills of residents
Jacobson & Ackerman, 1992	38 small group homes (Mean = 7 residents)	22%[b]	Public versus private operation Resident disability level

[a] 88 of the facilities studied were vocational; 164 were residential (mean size was not reported).
[b] 6 other variables were included but did not make unique contributions to explaining variability in tenure.

Table 2. Single State Multiple Regression Studies of Individual-Level Turnover

Authors	Subjects	R^2	Variables Contributing to Prediction of Variance
Askvig & Vassiliou, 1991	96 current and former supervisors and direct support workers in one regional residential and vocational agency	41%[a]	Monthly income Age
Bachelder & Braddock, 1994	42 direct support workers with less than 6 months' tenure selected from 120 direct support workers in 120 small (16 or fewer residents) homes	40%	Informal co-worker support
Hatton & Emerson, 1993	64 full-time direct support workers in a residential setting	41%[b]	Satisfaction with self-development Satisfaction with income Commitment to working in community services Satisfaction with training Participation in decision making Support from supervisors Job feedback Job variety Amount of interaction with clients
Razza, 1993	236 direct support workers in 9 private New Jersey agencies	61%[c]	Agreement of job with personal values and goals Burnout Satisfaction with supervisor Employment history Current job satisfaction Intention to quit

[a] This study predicted length of time on the job.
[b] This study used propensity to leave as the dependent variable.
[c] This study used a path analysis to identify factors associated with current employees' staying or leaving after 6 months.

Table 3. National Multiple Regression Studies of Facility-Level Turnover

Authors	Subjects	R^2	Variables Contributing to Prediction of Variance
Braddock & Mitchell, 1992	618 private agencies (Mean = 15 residents)	8%[a]	Average wage Starting wage Health benefits Direct care ratio Per diem Level of mental retardation Unionization Facility size Facility age ICF-MR certification Hours of in-service training
Lakin & Bruininks, 1981	73 small private residences (1 to 64 person)	9%	Starting salary (indexed by average per capita income) Number of direct support workers employed in facility
Larson & Lakin, 1992	101 small group homes (6 or fewer residents)	7%	Number of direct support workers Using shift versus live-in workers

[a] Descriptions of this study did not indicate which variables made unique contributions to the prediction of turnover.

variance accounted for was much higher when individual characteristics were the predictor variables than when agency or environmental variables were used. These analyses did not include variables such as job satisfaction, job commitment, or support, although a separate analysis of the association of general job satisfaction and satisfaction with various aspects of direct service work was included in the Lakin and Bruininks (1981) study.

The use of statistical procedures to examine more than one variable at a time has contributed to the quality of the developmental disabilities literature on staff turnover, allowing preliminary study of the relative importance of several variables. Still several major issues remain unresolved. First, while most existing studies have examined turnover in institutions or in large community settings, fewer have focused on small community settings (major exceptions are listed on Tables 1 through 4). Additionally, while most direct support workers who leave do so within 12 months of being hired (Braddock & Mitchell, 1992), only Bachelder and Braddock (1994) focused specifically on variables influencing turnover for newly hired direct support workers. Second, while most studies used a facility-level analysis, studies using an individual level of analysis predicted more of the variability in turnover. More research needs to include individual-level variables that can be applied to recruitment and retention interventions. Third, existing studies have been atheoretical and loosely linked to an existing body of literature (e.g., tend to use different sets of

Table 4. National Studies of Turnover Using an Individual Level of Analysis

Authors	Subjects	R^2	Variables Contributing to Prediction of Variance
Lakin & Bruininks, 1981	224 direct support workers in private residences (all sizes)	22%[a,b]	Care person age Years lived in county Length of employment Characteristics of the treatment environment Live-in status Family also living in Special training for the job Accepting the job for professional reasons
Larson & Lakin, 1992	48 direct support workers in (1-6 person) homes	41%[c]	Highest education level No previous course work in mental retardation Salary as % of area average per capita income

[a] This statistic is Wilk's Lambda from a discriminant analysis of stayers versus leavers over a 1-year follow-up.

[b] In a separate analysis 9% of the variability in staying or leaving was accounted for by 6 job satisfaction variables.

[c] This study used intended length of stay as the dependent variable.

variables). Excepting Bachelder and Braddock (1994), Hatton and Emerson (1993), and Razza (1993), there have not been systematic attempts to build or test models of turnover within the developmental disabilities literature. Finally, most studies use cross-sectional approaches (Jacobson & Ackerman, 1992; Lakin & Bruininks, 1981; and Razza, 1993, are the major exceptions). Longitudinal studies are needed to make stronger inferences about reliable predictors of turnover.

Studies of Turnover in the Personnel Psychology Literature

More than 1,500 articles have been published in the last 100 years on personnel turnover based on studies in business, manufacturing and service industries, the military, and other occupations (Bluedorn, 1982; Muchinsky & Morrow, 1980; Price, 1989; Staw, 1980). Researchers have identified hundreds of variables related to turnover, developed several comprehensive models of the turnover process, tested the accuracy of those models, and conducted comprehensive meta-analytical analyses of key variables. Unlike the developmental disabilities literature, which focuses heavily on facility-level variables to predict turnover, the personnel psychology literature focuses heavily on individual-level variables related to turnover. Much of that literature is highly instructive of potentially beneficial directions for personnel studies in developmental disabilities.

Since Porter and Steers' (1973) seminal

literature review recommended that future research examine the interactive influence of variables on the turnover process, several models to explain the turnover process have been developed and tested (e.g., Arnold & Feldman, 1982; Bluedorn, 1982; Hom & Griffeth, 1991; Jackofsky, 1984; Michaels & Spector, 1982; Mobley, et al., 1979; Mobley, et al., 1978; Muchinsky & Morrow, 1980; Price, 1977; Price & Mueller, 1986; Saks, 1994; Steers & Mowday, 1981; Stumpf & Hartman, 1984). In all, these models incorporate more than 65 different variables. Some variables appear in only one or two models, but many models share variables. Among the variables appearing in three or more models are employee characteristics such as age, tenure, and family size; work-related characteristics such as job expectations, job satisfaction, organizational commitment, job performance, job search intent and activities, and intentions to stay or leave; labor market conditions such as alternate job availability, unemployment rate, and national and local economic conditions; employer characteristics such as number of employees and organizational structure; and finally job characteristics such as benefits, supervisory style, and job duties. Tests of these models, including some using sophisticated methods (e.g., Hom, et al., 1992) have confirmed the importance of many of these variables in explaining the turnover process. However, this testing does not clear up which model is most useful or contained the most powerful set of variables.

Table 5. Variables Included in Three Turnover Models

Arnold & Feldman (1982)	Bluedorn (1982)	Michaels and Spector (1982)
Age	Demographic characteristics (race, sex, age, education, length of service, etc.)	Age
Tenure		Salary level, job level and tenure
	Expectations	Pre-employment expectations
		Perceived job characteristics
	The organization experienced (centralization, formalization, differentiation, technology, communication, innovation, conflict, etc.)	Leadership consideration
Job satisfaction	Job satisfaction	Job satisfaction
Organizational commitment	Organizational commitment	Organizational commitment
Intent to search for alternatives	Job search	
Perceived job security	Environmental opportunity	Perceived alternative employment
	Intent to leave	Intent to quit

These models were primarily designed to explain the sequence through which people who decide to leave go. However, they also provide a theoretical basis for identifying variables that explain variability in turnover rates. Probably the most tested models of the turnover process were developed by Mobley, et al. (1978), and Mobley, et al. (1979). Those models include many variables related to turnover in meta-analytic studies. The Hom & Griffeth (1991) study provides evidence of the validity of the Mobley, et al. (1978), model for describing the turnover process. Unlike most contemporary turnover models, however, the Mobley models do not include organizational commitment, a variable of substantial importance in explaining turnover (e.g., Kline & Peters, 1991). Organizational commitment is "the relative strength of an individual's identification with and involvement in a particular organization," and is characterized by a strong belief in and acceptance of the organization's goals and values, a willingness to exert considerable effort on behalf of the organization, and a strong desire to maintain membership in the organization (Mowday, et al., 1982, p. 226). Models proposed by Arnold & Feldman (1982), Bluedorn (1982), and Michaels & Spector (1982) share most variables with these other models and include organizational commitment (see Table 5). The Michaels and Spector (1982) model modifies Mobley, et al. (1979), specifically by adding the organizational commitment variable. These models provide a useful basis for selecting variables in studies of turnover rates.

Analysis of the predictors of turnover has been enhanced by 14 meta-analytical studies conducted since 1984 looking at various combinations of variables that could predict turnover (Bycio, et al., 1990; Carston & Spector, 1987; Cohen, 1993; Cotton & Tuttle, 1986; Hom, et al., 1992; Irvine & Evans, 1995; Mathieu & Zajac, 1990; McEvoy & Cascio, 1987; Mitra, et al., 1992; Randall, 1990; Steel & Ovalle, 1984; Tett & Meyer, 1993; Wanous,

et al., 1992; Williams & Livingstone, 1994). Only six variables were associated with turnover in more than one meta-analysis: organizational commitment (6 analyses, corrected *mean r* = -.23 to -.38); overall job satisfaction (6 analyses, corrected *mean r* = -.12 to -.28); intent to stay or leave (5 analyses, corrected *mean r* = .32 to .50); performance (3 analyses, corrected *mean r* = -.16 to -.28) and met expectations (2 analyses, corrected *mean r* = .33). Other variables were examined in one meta-analysis and had moderate to low significant correlations with turnover including: work satisfaction, pay satisfaction, satisfaction with supervisors, satisfaction with co-workers, satisfaction with promotion, accession rate, union presence, pay, role clarity, age, tenure, gender, biographical data, education, number of dependents, aptitude and ability, absence, thoughts of quitting, employment perceptions, unemployment rate, search intentions, and probability of getting an alternative job. In general these meta-analytic studies confirmed the importance of most of the variables in the turnover models described here.

Issues in Applying the Personnel Literature to Developmental Disabilities

In using the personnel psychology literature to guide personnel studies within agencies supporting persons with developmental disabilities, several lessons might be applied. First, studies must include individual-level analyses as well as facility-level analyses (e.g., Baysinger & Mobley, 1983; Campion, 1991; Muchinsky & Morrow, 1980). All of the turnover models reviewed earlier focused on predicting whether an individual employee would choose to stay or leave. In addition, in the developmental disabilities literature, research using individual level variables consistently explained more of the variations in turnover rates than research at the facility level.

A second lesson of the literature is that

Table 6. Strategies to Address Recruitment and Retention Challenges

During the Application Process
- Selection strategies
- Recruitment sources
- Recruitment strategies: realistic job previews

During Organizational Entry
- Orientation strategies
- Initial socialization

During Organizational Socialization
- Peer mentoring
- Competency-based staff training

Ongoing Strategies
- Enhancing the status of and opportunities available to direct support workers
- Developing links with higher education
- Staff development for supervisors
- Ongoing internal evaluation of efforts

those who are fired or otherwise left unavoidably should be separated from those who chose to leave (Abelson & Baysinger, 1984; Campion, 1991). Measures of voluntariness can be obtained by asking the employee who left (Campion, 1991). A further refinement measures the functionality or impact of the turnover for the organization by asking first-line supervisors to judge whether they would rehire a person who has left (Dalton, et al., 1982).

A third lesson relates to the need to attend to differences within the industries studied (e.g., general business, manufacturing industries, military settings, and service settings). While some personnel psychology literature is conducted in human service settings, such as nursing homes, other research subjects include professionals, such as MBAs in their first job after graduate school, army recruits, and commercial service industry employees. The wages, benefits, job conditions, employee characteristics, job expectations, and so forth may be very different from one group to another, and from those in settings supporting people with developmental disabilities. It should not, therefore, be assumed that variables associated with turnover in one industry or setting will necessarily apply directly to others.

The fourth lesson is that time is an important methodological component in the study of turnover. The selection of a time period for a study can greatly influence the statistical power of analysis procedures. The statistical procedures most often used in turnover research work best when the proportions of stayers and leavers are as close to 50% as possible (Bass & Ager, 1991; Huselid & Day, 1991; Kemery, et al., 1989; Steel & Griffeth, 1989; Steel, et al., 1990). When the proportion is not 50%, the total possible correlation between turnover and other variables is less than would be found if the split is 50-50 (Kemery, et al., 1989). This means that researchers should strive to select a time frame that will divide the stayers and leavers as close to 50% as possible. In residential settings for persons with developmental disabilities, this is sometime between 6 months and 12 months after hire (Bachelder & Braddock, 1994; Braddock & Mitchell, 1992; Ganju, 1979; Lakin & Bruininks, 1981).

Improving Personnel Practices to Address Recruitment and Retention Challenges

Most studies of personnel retention in developmental disabilities literature (and in the general personnel psychology literature as well) have focused on factors associated with staying or leaving as though research is an end in itself. While identifying factors associated with turnover is important, it is important to the extent that it contributes to identifying strategies that can reduce undesirable turnover. In recent years many techniques and recommendations have been forwarded to address recruitment and retention challenges. This review summarizes those identified in a thorough review of the developmental disabilities literature, and a selected sample of strategies discussed in the personnel psychology literature.

Strategies to address recruitment and retention challenges fall into four broad categories: prehire strategies, strategies for organizational entry, strategies for organizational socialization, and ongoing strategies. Table 6 provides an overview of recruitment and retention strategies in these categories.

During the Application Process

Several strategies can be implemented before a worker is hired. These are summarized here.

Selection Strategies

Selection is the process used by the organization to improve the matches between employee skills and potential, and organizational job requirements (Wanous, 1992). A mismatch between the employee's skills and the job requirements can lead to poor performance and termination of underqualified employees, or to dissatisfaction and voluntary quitting for an overqualified employee (Wanous, 1992). Strategies to improve selection processes include realistic work sample tests and simulations, assessment centers and simulations, and structured interviews. As an example of the latter, use of the Employee Reliability Inventory, a preinterview instrument, measuring freedom from substance abuse, courteous job performance, emotional maturity, conscientiousness, trustworthiness, long-term job commitment, and safe job performance, was associated with lower turnover rates and fewer work-related accidents among employees in a resort hotel/conference center (Borofsky, et al., 1993). The instrument was used to develop follow-up questions to be asked during interviews and reference checks. The goal of improving selection is to reduce the number of people to whom a job is offered to those most likely to do a good job for the organization.

Recruitment Sources

Recruitment is the process used by the organization to communicate with potential employees that a position is available, and to describe that position in a way that leads the potential employee to accept a job offered (Wanous, 1992). A mismatch between the employee's job wants and the organization's climate (the way things are done) can reduce satisfaction and organizational commitment, which could lead to voluntary quitting. Strategies to improve recruitment efforts include recruiting workers who heard about the job through a personal contact with either the agency or employees of the agency, developing networks of potential employees, working with school-to-work and welfare-to-work programs to target human services careers for their participants, and providing realistic information about the job to applicants before they take the job.

One tested recruitment strategy is the use of inside or informal sources to recruit new workers. Inside sources are referrals from sources that provide information not typically available to persons outside the company (Wanous, 1992). Examples of inside sources are rehires, referrals, and in-house notices targeted at current employees, volunteers, and friends of staff members. Outside sources are referrals from sources providing less specific information about the organization as a place to work (Wanous, 1992). Examples of outside sources include newspaper ads, employment agencies, and high school, technical college, and college placement offices. In a summary of 12 studies, job survival (the number of months a new hire stays in the organization) was 24% higher for employees recruited using inside sources than for employees using outside sources (Wanous, 1992). The benefit was greater among agencies that had high turnover rates. Another study found workers who heard about the job through multiple informal sources, those who were rehired, and those who learned about the company through a clinical rotation had the most prehire knowledge while those recruited through walking in or through advertisements had the least prehire knowledge. Increased prehire knowledge was associated with lower turnover among 234 nursing applicants ($r = -.25, p < .05$) (Williams, et al., 1993). Despite the effectiveness of inside recruitment sources, this same study found that 45% of new hires were walk-ins or had heard about the job through an advertisement, while only 25% of new hires had heard about the company through multiple informal sources, rehiring, or clinical rotations. Other recent studies also confirm the benefits of using informal recruitment sources in increasing information about and commitment to the job, improving the extent to which prehire expectations are met, and improving job survival (Saks, 1994; Taylor, 1994). The Saks (1994) study included a path analysis showing that both recruitment source and information provided by the organization were significant contributors to job survival.

It is unlikely that simply using inside recruitment sources will be sufficient to address current recruitment and retention challenges for direct support workers in community services for persons with developmental disabilities. With the current turnover rates, high vacancy rates, and continued industry growth, it is also necessary to identify and implement strategies using external recruitment to attract more workers to the field. Recruitment sources may need to be cultivated using medium- and long-term strategies to enlarge and stabilize the direct support workforce (Levy, et al., 1988). Short-term recruitment strategies, such as posting help-wanted advertisements, are the most common strategies used. Medium-term

strategies, such as cultivating relationships with career and placement resources through mailings of job listings, and long-term strategies, such as networking with area high school guidance counselors and postsecondary training programs, may be a key to recruiting high quality candidates over the long-term (Levy, et al., 1988).

Historically, the direct support workforce in community services has been drawn from young adult women with at least some postsecondary education (Larson, et al., 1994). Adequate supplies of workers in the future will likely depend on tapping new sources of potential recruits including older or displaced workers and people from groups that have traditionally experienced high unemployment rates (e.g., young mothers, unskilled workers, and high school drop-outs). To recruit these workers it will be necessary to join with community education and training programs, such as school-to-work initiatives, welfare-to-work initiatives, postsecondary education programs, "tech prep" initiatives, and vocational or technical programs, to recruit and train new direct support workers (Hewitt & Larson, 1997). Such recruitment efforts will require developing marketing materials and information about the types of jobs available within the industry. Information about jobs can also effectively be communicated by providing on-the-job experiences to students enrolled in "tech prep," school-to-work, and other internship programs. The value of these types of recruitment strategies, especially if they include an internship (whether paid or not), is that they provide good information about what to expect in the job. Previous experience, whether through internships or former jobs, is clearly associated with lower turnover rates (cf., Balfour & Neff, 1993; Lakin & Bruininks, 1981). Another way to provide experience is to develop and use a pool of screened and trained temporary workers who can fill vacancies due to illness, vacation, or vacancy. One such pool developed collaboratively by several provider agencies in Multnomah County, Oregon, was used to identify workers who were good matches who were then hired by the agencies they began in as relief workers (Orcutt, 1989).

There have been few studies of recruitment strategies in human service settings. In one study, 23 recruitment strategies (see Table 7) were evaluated by 320 directors of occupational therapy units (Smith, et al., 1995). Of those 23 strategies, the most commonly used strategies were referrals from current staff members, professional development opportunities, and newspaper advertisements. The strategies rated as most effective were providing a competitive salary, providing student internships, and sponsoring student training. Those rated as least effective strategies were telephone recruitment, career days, and open houses.

Table 7. Recruitment Strategies Used for Occupational Therapists*

Type of Strategy	Examples (rated effectiveness)[a]
Salary and compensation	Competitive salary (4.03) Student sponsorships (3.70) Sign-on bonus (3.38) Relocation expenses (3.27) Paid interview expenses (2.85)
Work experiences (prehire)	Student internships (3.97) Clinical rotations (3.47) Student supervision (2.85)
Benefits	Professional development (3.59) Flexible work schedules (3.55) On-site child care (3.02)
Work experiences (posthire)	Clinical (career) ladder (3.39) Program development (3.12) Conducting research (2.48) Direct recruitment (inside sources) Referrals from staff members (3.61) Telephone contacts (2.83) Contacting previous applicants (2.25)
Advertisement	Professional journal advertisements (3.17) Newspaper advertisements (2.81) Licensure listings (2.48)
Direct recruitment (outside sources)	Career days (2.46) Job fairs (2.24) Open houses (2.10)

* Based on a study by Smith, et al. (1995). Within each category strategies are listed according to their rated effectiveness for recruiting occupational therapists.
[a] 1 = least effective, 5 = most effective

Recruitment Strategies: Realistic Job Previews

Realistic job previews (RJPs) are a third promising strategy that can be implemented during the application process. Realistic job previews are grounded on the theory that unmet expectations held by newcomers about important aspects of the job and organization cause low job satisfaction and low organizational commitment. Low satisfaction and organizational commitment, in turn, cause newcomers to quit (Wanous, 1989, 1992). Realistic job previews use strategies such as audiovisuals, booklets, oral presentations, interviews, and work sample tests to present to outsiders pertinent information about the job and the organization without distortion before a decision is made about whether to take the job (Wanous, 1992). Realistic job previews are used to reduce the number of applicants who would accept a job offer to just those who wish to work under the conditions (both positive and negative) described in the RJP. This reduces quitting by new hires who start the job only to find out that it is not what they expected the job to be.

A study of the effectiveness of RJPs for workers in an institution serving people with developmental disabilities found that use of a written RJP was associated with modest but statistically significant increases in the mean length of service for newly hired direct support workers (Zaharia & Baumeister, 1981). Meta-analyses of the effects of realistic job previews across several studies provide a clearer picture of the potential usefulness of this technique (Breaugh, 1983; McEvoy & Cascio, 1985; Premack & Wanous, 1985). In one meta-analysis, RJPs improved retention rates (the rates at which new hires remain on the job for a specific length of time) by from 9% to 17% (McEvoy & Cascio, 1985). In another meta-analysis, RJPs increased retention by 12% for agencies with annual retention rates of 50% and by 24% for agencies with retention rates of 20% (Premack & Wanous, 1985). RJPs also lowered initial job expectations while increasing self-selection, organizational commitment, job satisfaction, and performance. In short, RJPs make a difference, one that is larger for agencies with higher turnover rates.

Wanous (1989) identified and discussed several considerations involved in variations in the design and implementation of RJPs. Those considerations included:

- whether it should be developed to reduce existing turnover problems or to prevent potential problems,
- whether the organizational analysis used to develop the content should be structured or unstructured,
- whether the content should be descriptive or judgmental,
- whether it should be extensive and cover broadly information needed by many recruits, or intensive and focus on just a few key points for a specific group of employees,
- whether the RJP should be highly or just moderately negative,
- whether a written or audio-visual medium should be used,
- whether actors or actual employees should be used in filming the RJP,
- whether the RJP should be used early or late in the organizational entry process,
- whether the RJPs should be introduced as a pilot study, or as a permanent component of the normal recruiting practice, and
- whether the results of using RJPs should be studied and disseminated.

Two studies have examined the impact of design issues on the effectiveness of RJPs. A longitudinal study examined the issue of how negative the RJP should be. This study of 533 U.S. Army trainees compared enhancement previews (designed to enhance overly pessimistic expectations) with reduction previews (designed to reduce overly optimistic expectations; Meglino, et al., 1988). Results showed that rainees exposed to both previews had significantly lower turnover, those exposed only to the reduction preview had significantly higher turnover, and RJPs were more effective in reducing turnover among more intelligent and committed trainees. In a second study of 1,117 applying correctional officers (of whom 358 accepted positions), a realistic job preview that lowered expectations reduced the rate of job acceptances among those who had previous exposure to the job, but increased the rate of job acceptances among applicants with no previous exposure (Meglino, et al., 1993). Also, among applicants with previous job experience, those who saw the job preview had lower retention rates during probation, but higher retention rates after probation than those who did not see the job preview. The implication is that realistic job previewing techniques may not be equally effective among different types of applicants.

Several reports of how realistic job preview strategies could be used have appeared in recent years. One study of home health aides and homemakers described an assessment process in which workers reported they did not like to do housework, paperwork was excessive and not clearly explained, mailing costs to turn in paperwork was unreasonable, and communication between the worker and the agency was inadequate (Ditson, 1994). In response, the agency restructured its interviewing process and job description to make sure recruits had a realistic picture of the work they would be doing. They also streamlined paperwork processes and provided additional training on how to complete it. They made the orientation process more intentional to provide a clear understanding of the process from beginning to end. They added a peer mentor system in which new hires were assigned a person to shadow as they began their job. Finally, they established a peer recognition committee and a system for distributing important information to

workers. These practices reduced turnover among home health aides from 43% to 40% and for homemakers from 90% to 81%. In addition, the number of home health aides who continued to work after orientation increased from 63% to 75% and the number of homemakers who continued to work after orientation increased from 38% to 68%. These differences were not tested to see if they reached statistical significance. This study illustrates the usefulness of completing an agency-specific assessment related to job content and staff reactions and developing specific RJP interventions in response. But the study's relatively modest effects on turnover demonstrate that prehire strategies alone will seldom adequately resolve turnover problems.

During Organizational Entry

Orientation Strategies

Orientation programs are designed to help newcomers cope with the stress of starting a new job. A model for conducting orientation called Realistic Orientation Programs for new Employee Stress (ROPES) was developed by Wanous (1992). This model suggests that stress can be reduced by:

- including realistic information about initial stresses,
- providing general support and assurance (in small groups or one-to-one),
- demonstrating coping skills including: dealing directly with the stress, modifying ways you think about stress, reappraising the situation (e.g., you are not a bad person because a consumer hit you; everyone makes some mistakes at the beginning), and managing the symptoms of stress (e.g., exercise, relaxation, deep breathing),
- discussing the examples and effects of suggestions provided,
- rehearsing using the modeled strategies,
- teaching self-management of thoughts and feelings, and

- targeting information about stressors to specific newcomers to whom they apply.

Realistic orientation programs are designed to help newcomers want to stay in the organization (Wanous, 1992). The importance of assisting workers with stress management was confirmed in a New York survey of more than 600 direct support workers, 44% of whom identified stress management as their top training need (Ebenstein & Gooler, 1993).

Initial Socialization

Organizational socialization is a process involving social learning of new roles, norms and values, and conflicts. Organizational socialization unfolds over time as newcomers change to conform to the organization (Wanous, 1992). Van Maanen and Schein (1979) describe organizational socialization as the process by which one is taught and learns the ropes of a particular organizational role. They postulate that socialization, although continuous throughout one's career within an organization, is more intense and problematic for a member (and others) just before and just after a particular boundary passage such as starting a new job (Van Maanen & Schein, 1979).

Louis (1980) discusses two stages of socialization: (a) anticipatory socialization, in which recruits anticipate their experiences and develop expectations about their life in the organization; and (b) encounter socialization, in which newcomers' anticipations are tested against the reality of their new work experiences. Coping with the differences between expectations and experiences occupy the newcomer for the first 6 to 10 months on a new job. In Louis' (1980) model, three aspects of the process of initial socialization or organizational entry are noted: (a) change—objective differences in major features between the old and new settings; (b) contrast—person-specific perceptions of salient features of the new environment; and (c) surprise—the difference between an individual's expectations

and subsequent experiences. The process of making sense of surprises involves processing past experiences, presuppositions and purposes, others' interpretations, and local interpretation schemes to develop a new cognitive script to decide how to move ahead. The challenge of supporting newcomers is to give them information needed to balance the information from these sources to make meaning from the surprises.

Socialization practices differ along six dimensions: collective versus individual, formal versus informal, sequential versus variable, fixed versus variable, serial versus disjunctive, and investiture versus divestiture (Van Maanen & Schein, 1979).

- Collective socialization refers to taking a group of recruits through a common set of experiences; individual socialization refers to processing recruits individually in isolation from one another.
- Formal socialization occurs when a newcomer is segregated from the more experienced members while being put through a set of specifically tailored experiences; informal socialization does not separate a newcomer's role, and does not differentiate between recruits and more experienced members.
- Sequential socialization refers to the degree to which the organization specifies a given sequence of discrete identifiable steps leading to the target role; random socialization refers to a sequence of steps that is unknown, ambiguous or continually changing.
- Fixed socialization processes provide precise information about how long it will take to complete the process; variable socialization gives few clues about when to expect a boundary change.
- Serial socialization refers to a process in which newcomers follow in the footsteps of experienced members and are groomed for the role by them; disjunctive socialization occurs when there are no immediate predecessors to follow, and

where role models are not available to inform newcomers about how to perform.

- Finally, investiture socialization ratifies and documents the viability and usefulness of the personal characteristics the newcomer brings to the organization; divestiture socialization processes deny and attempt to strip away selected personal characteristics of a new recruit.

Jones (1986) classified these six dimensions according to whether the socialization was institutionalized or individualized. He argued that institutionalized socialization tactics involve collective, formal, sequential, fixed, serial, and investiture socialization, while individualized socialization tactics involve individual, informal, random, variable, disjunctive, and divestiture socialization strategies. He hypothesized that institutionalized socialization tactics will be negatively related to role conflict, role ambiguity and intention to quit, and positively related to job satisfaction and commitment. He developed a scale to measure socialization tactics and tested his hypotheses on 102 MBAs. The resulting canonical function suggested that institutionalized socialization patterns were negatively related to role conflict, role ambiguity, and intent to quit and positively related to job satisfaction and commitment (Jones, 1986). This research was replicated and extended by Allen & Meyer (1990). Using Jones' Socialization Tactics Questionnaire, they found that fixed and investiture socialization tactics explained a significant proportion of variability in organizational commitment at 6 months' tenure, but that by 12 months' tenure, only investiture strategies contributed significantly to variability in organizational commitment (Allen & Meyer, 1990). They concluded that agencies that wished to enhance organizational commitment (and possibly lower turnover) should use investiture socialization strategies.

The research on socialization strategies was extended into the developmental disabilities literature by Bachelder and Braddock (1994). Their factor analysis of the socialization tactics scale produced two factors, informal co-worker support and role clarity, for workers in small residential settings. They reported that informal co-worker support was significantly negatively correlated with turnover among direct support workers with less than 6 months of experience (Bachelder & Braddock, 1994). Elements of co-worker support were: co-workers go out of their way to help a new staff member adjust to the job, newcomers are able to gain a clear understanding of the work role by observing co-workers, experienced staff members see advising or training newcomers as one of their main job responsibilities, experienced staff members provide guidance to newcomers about how to perform the job, and the training process expands and builds on job knowledge gained in previous training. They recommended that managers develop intervention strategies during the initial employment period to encourage co-worker support.

The need for and importance of co-worker support is implied in a study of 693 direct support workers in New York City. In that study 26% of workers who had less than 7 months' tenure on the job reported dissatisfaction with a negative social atmosphere compared with only 12% of workers with 7 to 12 months' tenure (Ebenstein & Gooler, 1993). This suggests that either workers who were dissatisfied with the social atmosphere left during the first six months, or the atmosphere was less negative once a worker had been in the organization awhile. A study of socialization practices found that the most frequently used and the most helpful socialization practices for recent business school graduates were a buddy relationship with a more senior co-worker, the initial supervisor, and daily interactions with peers while working (Louis, et al., 1983). Intent to stay in the organization was significantly correlated with the helpfulness of daily interactions with peers while working, support from the initial supervisor, extended off-site training, and business trips.

A separate longitudinal study of 248 new hires in a range of career fields including business, engineering, sales, management, education, medicine, social services, and others found that the negative outcomes (turnover intentions, low organizational commitment, and low job satisfaction) associated with unmet expectations can be improved by high-quality interactions between new hires and supervisors (leader-member exchange) and by high-quality interactions between new hires and members of the work group (team-member exchange) (Major, et al., 1995). These studies confirm the importance of the supervisor and other team members in the initial socialization of newcomers.

During Organizational Socialization

Organizational socialization continues well into the first year of employment. Several strategies have been identified as assisting with socialization during and after orientation. One line of research emphasizes that socialization is not only affected by organizational initiatives, but also by the initiative of the newcomer. In a longitudinal study of newcomers, controlling for differences soon after entry and for information received in other ways, information seeking by the newcomer was associated with increases in task mastery, role clarity, and social integration at 6 months (Morrison, 1993). By implication, organizations that promote and reinforce information seeking can enhance individual initiative and contribute to organizational socialization. Two other strategies useful during the first year of employment are peer mentoring and competency-based staff training.

Peer Mentoring

Peer mentoring strategies link new employees with more senior direct support workers to help in socialization to the job and in developing or practicing specific skills needed for the job (Hewitt, Larson, Ebenstein & Rose, 1996). Peer mentoring can reduce isolation of direct support workers and increase supports. It can also allow supervisors to delegate the tasks of answering routine questions about the job. Peer mentors benefit by developing a broader understanding of the work and of their co-workers. In one study about half (45%) of newly hired business graduates reported that a mentor or sponsor was available to them (Louis, et al., 1983). Mentors ranked fourth in how helpful they were to new hires after the helpfulness of peers, supervisors, and senior co-workers. The helpfulness of mentors to new employees was significantly correlated to job satisfaction ($r = .23, p < .05$) but not to organizational commitment or tenure intention. In a New York study, 12 of 24 agencies reported using peer mentoring with at least some staff members (Ebenstein & Gooler, 1993). Of those agencies 58% mentor employees once a week, and 33% said their mentoring efforts were extremely or usually effective. Reasons for problems with mentoring programs included lack of advancement opportunities for those mentored (88%), protégée leaves and takes the skills with him or her (88%), not enough time to mentor properly (33%), and too much resentment by others not being mentored (33%) (Ebenstein & Gooler, 1993).

Other studies of peer mentoring have reported positive results. A study of a mentoring program for 120 beginning teachers in Los Angeles documented an increased retention rate from 78% to 95% for the first 3 years on the job (Colbert & Wolff, 1992). The project had three major components. The first was establishing teams of two to four beginning teachers and one lead teacher at each school. These teams kept a journal documenting a minimum of 60 hours of meetings covering a range of specified and nonspecified topics each school year. The teams were monitored and supported through visitations to the school sites, individual meetings and regular phone conversations with participants, analysis of journal entries, and formative evaluation questionnaires. The second component was training for lead teachers in methods of classroom observation and coaching. Those lead teachers provided support and feedback to project participants. The third component was joint enrollment of both beginning and lead teachers in a series of credited university courses and 1-day retreats on topics that many beginning teachers find challenging. Costs ranged from $3,000 to $4,000 per participant per year.

Another study examined the effect of giving newcomers a mentor for information gathering during early socialization (Ostroff & Kozlowski, 1993). In this study mentors were not peers but employees at a higher level in the organization and someone other than an immediate supervisor. Mentors helped by taking the individual under their wings even though they were not formerly required to do so. That study found that mentors were used most to provide information about role and organizational features such as politics, procedures, and policies. Newcomers with mentors had more information about their roles and the organization than those who did not have mentors. When newcomers did not have mentors, they used co-workers to gather more information about the job than did newcomers with mentors.

Competency-Based Staff Training

Training of new direct support workers is considered important, because it is a direct regulatory mandate for most human services agencies (Larson, et al., 1994); it is considered a key element in achieving higher quality services (Alpha Group, 1990; Fiorelli, et al., 1982); it provides the opportunity to learn critical job functions, develop new skills, and cope with job roles (Camp, et al., 1986); and it develops attitudes and skills among employees that affect the quality of life for individuals with developmental disabilities (Jones, et al., 1981). A study of 1,736 new hires in different organizations suggested that workers who complete more weeks of training ($m = 4.5$ weeks of training for workers who stayed more than 7 months) had significantly lower turnover than workers in agencies with fewer weeks of training ($m = 1.9$ weeks of training for workers who voluntarily resigned) (Wanous, et al., 1979). Voluntary leavers also were less likely to receive informal job training (20% for leavers vs. 43% for stayers).

Ostroff and Kozlowski (1992) identified characteristics of effective training during socialization. They found that newcomers sought information about their tasks (e.g., duties, assignments, priorities, use of equipment, handling routine problems) and roles (e.g., boundaries of authority and responsibility, expectations and appropriate behaviors for the position) from observing how others do things, trial and error, and communication with their supervisors and co-workers, and that they sought information about their group (e.g., co-worker interaction, group norms and values) and organization (politics, power, values of organization, mission, leadership style) from observing others. Significantly more knowledge was gained from observation and trying things out than from interaction with supervisors or co-workers or from reading in manuals. Ostroff and Kozlowsky (1992) also found that obtaining more information from supervisors was correlated with higher satisfaction and commitment and lesser desire to leave the organization. Finally, individuals who believed they possessed more knowledge were more satisfied, committed, and adjusted and less likely to want to leave the organization. These results support the need to provide hands-on opportunities to develop and demonstrate new skills rather than simply talk about them, and to involve supervisors in providing the information needed by new workers about effective job performance.

Ongoing Strategies

Enhancing the Status and Opportunities Available to Direct Support Workers

Although direct support workers constitute a substantial majority of the developmental disabilities workforce, they do not have professional status, and they have the least power and visibility among all workers in the field (Hewitt, O'Nell, & Larson, 1996). Recently attempts have been made to identify the problems caused by this circumstance and potential solutions. The 1995 conference Listening to New Hampshire's Caregivers, cosponsored by a consortium of public agencies, provided direct support workers an opportunity to share ideas and concerns (Covert, 1995). Direct support workers made several suggestions for improving work environments. Workers suggested the need to increase respect both for people with disabilities and their direct support workers. Specific suggestions included:

- having administrators spend time in direct support work to get a taste of the reality and issues for both consumers and staff,
- respecting direct support workers the same way professionals are respected,
- increasing efforts to survey direct support workers about their work,
- asking the people being served what they would like their staff to learn, and
- holding regular meetings between families and direct support workers.

Direct support workers also suggested including direct support workers in decision making. Specific suggestions included:

- providing easier access to program administrators (e.g., through open forums),
- inviting direct support workers to serve on all agency committees and teams,
- promoting team building within the agency, and using teams to solve prob-

lems and to generate innovative suggestions,
- including direct support workers in meetings concerning the agency's budget,
- holding regular meetings to obtain input from direct support workers regarding what is important to provide quality support for consumers, and
- providing backup coverage so direct support workers can participate in Individual Service Planning meetings.

Finally, direct support workers suggested increasing training opportunities for direct support workers, and focusing on the quality of each individual's life.

Other strategies to enhance the recognition and support of direct support workers include targeting markets using popular media; providing opportunities for direct support workers to influence agency and public policy, and the development of services and supports; defining, supporting, and acknowledging direct support worker competence; and developing specific opportunities for workers to gather with their colleagues to exchange ideas and receive mutual support (Hewitt & Larson, 1997; Hewitt, Larson, Ebenstein, & Rose, 1996). These recommendations, with their heavy emphasis on respecting direct support personnel and the importance of their work and the skills required to perform it well, suggest many interventions that may improve working conditions, job satisfaction, and commitment of these workers. The potential for effectiveness of such approaches is supported by a meta-analysis study that found that job enrichment strategies to enhance decision-making authority, task variety, and autonomy reduced turnover rates by 17% among persons in a wide variety of work roles (McEvoy & Cascio, 1985).

Respect and interpersonal issues within the organization also have been identified in several other studies. A study of 34 certified nursing assistants found that while 24%

reportedly left their position because they got another job, 24% of leavers did so because of personal or staff conflicts (Gaddy & Bechtel, 1995). Direct support workers reported that the least liked parts about the job included negative social atmosphere (e.g., lack of communication, lack of help or cooperation, not getting along with others; 20%) and supervision and management (e.g., poor supervision, bad management, agency politics, favoritism; 17%) (Ebenstein & Gooler, 1993). Even human services supervisors identify and acknowledge the importance of respect and work relationships. A study of 329 directors of occupational therapy programs rated work relationships, the nature of supervision, work hours, and salary and compensation as the most effective retention strategies (Smith, et al., 1995) (See Table 8).

Table 8. Retention Strategies Used for Occupational Therapists

Type of Strategy	Examples (rated effectiveness)[a]
Work relationships	Interpersonal staff member relationships (4.17)
Nature of supervision	Supportive environment (4.16) Supervision and feedback (3.72) Employee appraisals (3.27)
Work hours	Flexible work hours (3.85) Part-time work hours (3.68) Job sharing (3.39)
Salary and compensation	Competitive salary (4.02) Length-of-stay incentives (3.16)
Recognition	Employee recognition (3.56)
Responsibility	Professional autonomy (3.81) Treatment of multiple conditions (3.58) Mentoring of students (3.14)
Facility and administration	Reputation of the facility (3.89) Patient-therapist ratio (3.59) Job security (3.52) Facility committee work (2.58)
Benefits	Paid professional memberships (3.09) On-site child care (2.96)
Advancement and growth	Continuing education (3.70) Career plan and model (3.52) Advancement opportunities (3.51) Research opportunities (2.52)

Based on a study by Smith, et al. (1995). Within each category strategies are listed according to their rated effectiveness for retaining occupational therapists.

[a] 1 = least effective, 5 = most effective

Developing Links With Higher Education

The Kennedy Fellows Mentoring Program provides scholarships and career mentoring to direct support workers enrolled for at least six credits in two New York colleges (Hewitt, Larson, & Ebenstein, 1996). This program encourages direct support workers to complete a 2-year degree, and helps them become eligible for promotions to positions with greater responsibility. Fifteen other states have federally funded Training Initiative Projects designed to identify, develop, and disseminate state-of-the-art training curricula; provide technical assistance and training to direct support workers, supervisors, agencies, consumers, and families; develop career ladder opportunities for direct support workers; complete training needs-assessments; and facilitate collaboration among key stakeholders regarding direct support issues (AAUAP, 1996). These projects reflect the growing national interest in and concern for developing, respecting, and supporting direct support workers. They also reflect examples of programs that can increase the visibility of careers in direct support work and help recruit new workers to the industry.

Staff Development for Supervisors

Several strategies to improve management practices to address personnel issues have been identified. A study of 968 publicly held firms throughout the U.S. with 100 employees or more found that 13 High Performance Work Practices (9 employee skill and organizational structure practices and 4 employee motivation practices) were associated with lower turnover rates and increased productivity (Huselid, 1995). Indicators of these High Performance Work Practices were:

Employee skills and organizational structure

- proportion of the workforce included in a formal information sharing program

(e.g., newsletter)
- proportion of the workforce whose job has been subjected to a formal job analysis
- proportion of non-entry-level jobs filled from within in recent years
- proportion of the workforce who are administered attitude surveys regularly
- proportion of the workforce who participate in Quality of Work Life programs, Quality Circles, and/or labor-management participation teams
- proportion of the workforce with access to company incentive plans, profit- sharing plans, and/or gain-sharing plans
- average number of hours of training received by a typical employee over the last 12 months
- proportion of the workforce with access to a formal grievance procedure and/or complaint resolution system
- proportion of the workforce administered an employment test before hiring

Employee motivation practices

- proportion of the workforce whose performance appraisals are used to decide their compensation
- proportion of the workforce receiving formal performance appraisals
- promotion decision rules [listed from least to most desirable] (a) seniority, (b) seniority among employees who meet a minimum merit requirement, (c) seniority only if merit is equal, (d) merit or performance rating alone
- number of qualified applicants per position for the five positions hired most frequently

Informing supervisors and managers in human service settings about these strategies, along with the other strategies identified in this review, and how to do them is an important part of addressing the recruitment and retention challenges we now face.

Other Strategies

The Ford Foundation sponsored a project that assembled a combination of interventions to address turnover among home health aides in 11 agencies in four cities (Feldman, 1993). The interventions consisted of basic and/or specialized supplemental training, professional and/or peer support and/or supervision, wage increments, supplemental benefits including health insurance, vacation and/or sick leave, increased predictability (guaranteed hours and/or full-time work), status enhancements (e.g., badges, uniforms, job titles), and promotions. One-year follow-up reviews found that all of the projects reduced turnover (differences ranged from 10% to 44% between participant and control turnover rates). Cities that used the most comprehensive interventions also had the largest decreases in turnover rates. Costs of the project ranged from $1.43 per hour per worker in the most comprehensive project (resulting in a 44% difference in turnover rates), to $0.09 per hour per worker for the least comprehensive project (resulting in a 10% difference in turnover rates).

Another recommendation for enhancing the direct support role is to improve pay and benefits for direct support workers. A study of 297 private firms in Georgia found that firms where benefits were a higher percent-age of the total labor cost and firms whose benefit packages were of higher quality experienced lower turnover rates (Bennett, et al., 1993). This was true after accounting for size, type of agency, rural location, gender, age, and racial composition of employees. When asked what could be done to make their job better, 33% of direct support workers responded more money or a raise (Ebenstein & Gooler, 1993).

A final strategy to address staffing shortages caused by turnover is to overhire and then prepare workers to fill vacancies that did not yet exist (Cardona & Bernreuter, 1996). Overhires reduced the costs associated with temporarily filling vacated nursing positions (either through overtime or by using temporary agencies) by hiring workers with no previous experience and training them to competence before a position was available. During the study 13 of 14 nurses hired under this program were hired for a licensed position; the remaining nurse was hired for an unlicensed position. The cost of hiring and training newcomers for 7 weeks in anticipation of a vacancy was less than half the cost of waiting until after the posi-tion was vacant to hire a person with 2 years of experience. The overhire strategy could be useful for agencies supporting people with developmental disabilities as well. Develop-ing a competency-based training system in which people are hired and promised a position but required to complete training while waiting for an opening has the potential advantages of increasing the skills of people who take new positions and decreasing overtime costs incurred because a vacancy cannot be filled right away.

Ongoing Evaluation of Efforts

Many strategies reviewed here have at least preliminary support for their effectiveness. However, further work is needed to identify the particular combination of strategies that are most effective for particular situations. An important part of this work involves ongoing data collection efforts among current and leaving staff members to identify specific recruitment and retention challenges facing individual agencies and to match those challenges with potential solutions. Exit questionnaires and periodic surveys of employees provide valuable information about the types of changes that may be helpful in reducing turnover rates and improving job satisfaction. One residen-tial treatment facility serving children used an annual interviewing process (using a 25-item structured interview) to assess changes needed to address problems identified by staff members. This process was associated with a decline in turnover rate from 70% at baseline to just over 40% after 3 years of implementation (McDonnell & Wilson-Simpson, 1994). A comprehensive assessment process that could be used across agencies to evaluate current status, to identify potentially useful intervention strategies, and to evaluate the effectiveness of those strategies is regularly needed.

Summary

For agencies supporting people with developmental disabilities recruitment and retention challenges are immense and growing. Addressing those challenges will require research that not only identifies variables associated with recruitment and retention challenges, but also can be used to identify effective strategies to address them. This study addresses these challenges by evaluating a comprehensive set of variables to assess their association with turnover rates, extending the literature on factors that influence newly hired direct support workers, and providing information that can be used to develop assessment and intervention strategies to improve recruitment and reduce retention problems.

CHAPTER 4
STUDY METHODOLOGY

This chapter describes the procedures used to identify and recruit study participants, the design of the study, the instruments and variable definitions used, the procedures followed as the study was completed, and the analysis plans developed prior to the initiation of the study to analyze the results and answer the research questions. Separate descriptions are provided for the methods used in Study 1: The Study of Facility-Level Recruitment and Retention Issues, and in Study 2: The Study of Newly Hired Direct Support Workers during their first 12 months after hire.

Population and Sample

Selection of Agencies

A three-stage stratified random sampling procedure was used to identify agencies for this study. In the first stage, all 36 agencies providing residential services to people in the Minnesota Longitudinal Study (Hayden, et al., 1996) were contacted. In addition, all of the Regional Treatment Centers (RTCs) operating State-Operated Community Services (SOCS) homes for people with developmental disabilities were contacted. This first stage sampled agencies that supported people with mental retardation who moved from Minnesota's RTCs since 1990.

In the second stage, the mailing list of the Association of Residential Resources in Minnesota (ARRM, a trade group for Minnesota residential providers) was used to identify agencies not represented in the Minnesota Longitudinal Study. Sixty-seven additional agencies were randomly selected in two rounds from the 92 agencies on the ARRM membership list.

In the third stage, a list of all Minnesota agencies identified by the Department of Human Services, Division for Persons with Developmental Disabilities, as providing ICF-MR or HCBS Waiver funded residential services was obtained. An additional 25 agencies were randomly selected from among the remaining 83 agencies on the combined ARRM and DHS agency lists.

In all, 128 of the 188 agencies providing residential services to people with mental retardation in Minnesota in 1993 were invited to participate in this study. The second and third stages sampled from the population of all agencies providing residential services to persons with developmental disabilities in Minnesota.

Administrators from the identified agencies received a letter and a brochure describing the study. A letter of support from the Association on Residential Resources in Minnesota was included with the initial recruitment letter. The agencies were contacted to provide more detailed information about the study, answer any questions, and determine if any of the homes within the agency met the selection criteria for the study.

All of the agencies in the Minnesota Longitudinal Study were initially considered eligible, but two agencies in the Minnesota Longitudinal Study that provided only institutional care were subsequently excluded. Agencies not in the Minnesota Longitudinal Study with at least one home that provided 24-hour support to six or fewer people with mental retardation were considered eligible. Of the 128 agencies screened, 94 (73%) were eligible based on these criteria. Administrators with at least one eligible home were invited to participate. A total of 83 of the 94 eligible agencies (88%) submitted a letter of agreement to participate.

Selection of Participating Homes

Homes for the study were also selected in a two-phase process. In the first phase, supervisors of all State-Operated Community Services (SOCS) homes from participating RTCs and supervisors of all homes in the Minnesota Longitudinal Study were invited to participate. Identified supervisors who supervised more than one SOCS home or more than one home from the Minnesota Longitudinal Study were asked to complete the full study for the first home that became eligible, and the facility-only study for any additional homes. Supervisors who were not able to devote the required time to completing full study were also invited to limit their participation by being only in the facility phase of the study. In this first phase, supervisors in 116 homes were invited to participate, 108 based on being part of the Minnesota Longitudinal Study and 8 based on being a SOCS home.

In the second phase, administrators from 50 agencies not in the Minnesota Longitudinal Study were asked to report how many of their homes provided 24-hour supports to six or fewer people with developmental disabilities. If only one home was eligible, that home was selected. If two or more homes within the agency met the selection criteria, one home was randomly selected from the eligible homes. For the first eight agencies selected in this second phase, participating homes were randomly selected from homes that supported six or fewer people, at least one being a person who moved from an RTC in 1990 or later. For the remaining 42 agencies, homes were randomly selected from among all homes with six or fewer people served by the agency. As in the first phase, supervisors who were not able to devote the required time to completing full study were invited to limit their participation by being only in the facility phase of the study. In this second phase, 50 homes were identified. In all, supervisors in 166 homes were identified as possible participants in the study (110 from Phase 1 and 50 from Phase 2).

Supervisor Recruitment

Agency administrators provided information on how to contact the on-site supervisor in each eligible home. Letters of introduction and project brochures were mailed to each supervisor. A follow-up phone call provided more detailed information and answers to questions raised by supervisors. Supervisors who agreed to participate received a supervisor consent form. When the signed consent was returned, a packet of instructions and surveys was delivered to the supervisor. If a supervisor from a home selected in the second phase declined to participate, the researcher, working with the agency administrator, randomly selected another eligible home from that agency. Supervisors in 143 of the 166 selected homes (86%) agreed to participate. Of the 23 homes that did not participate, supervisors in 7 homes agreed to participate but did not complete any surveys, and supervisors in 16 homes declined to participate. Supervisors in 33 homes (all from the first selection phase) supporting more than six people returned surveys but were excluded from this analysis. Of the 110 homes included in this analysis, 68 homes were selected in the first phase and 42 homes were selected in the second phase of supervisor recruitment.

Selection of Direct Support Workers

Participating supervisors provided materials to direct support participants for this study. Up to three new workers per home were eligible to participate. Eligible workers met the following standards:

- The direct support worker voluntarily consented to participate.
- The person was a primary provider of support, training, supervision, and personal assistance for persons with mental retardation in the home. The person spent at least 50% of his or her hours in direct support activity.

- The direct support worker was new to this home. People returning to work in the home after a paid or unpaid leave of absence were excluded.
- The person may have been new to the agency or may have previously worked in other homes in this agency.
- The person worked regularly scheduled shifts in the home named on the surveys. People who worked only "on-call" hours were excluded.
- The person must have been hired to work in the home listed on the survey.

Supervisors provided the consent form and a project brochure to all eligible new hires during orientation, or as early in their employment as possible. In both written and spoken instructions to the supervisors, the voluntary nature of the study was emphasized. Supervisors were instructed to save the materials for the next person if a new hire declined to participate. Additional information about new hires who declined to participate is not available. In all, supervisors reported asking 333 direct support workers to participate in the study. Of the workers approached about the study, 174 (52%) workers from 110 different homes agreed to participate and returned a consent form and one or more surveys to the researchers, 49 (15%) agreed to participate but did not return a consent form, and 110 (33%) declined to participate. Six direct support workers who returned consents and at least one survey were excluded because they neither left the home nor completed 12 months at the home before data collection for the study ended. One person who returned a consent form and a Time 1 survey was excluded because an exit survey was not available. This left a total of 167 study participants.

Research Design

Facility Study

Two facility surveys were completed by participating supervisors. The first survey was administered when the home entered the study. For homes still in the study at that point, the second survey was administered 12 months after the first survey was returned. The supervisor could choose to complete the survey by means of interview or by written response. The facility surveys requested information about facility characteristics, staffing patterns, general staff characteristics, recruitment and retention challenges, and characteristics of the people living in the home. A short form of the facility survey was used to gather basic information from supervisors unwilling or unable to complete the regular facility survey. Supervisors in 143 homes completed the Time 1 (baseline) survey, and supervisors in 101 of 108 homes still in the study at Time 2 completed the Time 2 (1 year after baseline) survey (94%). Among the 110 homes included in this analysis, facility Time 1 surveys were available for 110 homes, facility Time 2 surveys were available for 80 homes, and facility short surveys were available at Time 2 for 16 homes.

Direct Support Worker Study

Five surveys were administered to up to three newly hired direct support workers in each home. The first survey was completed at hire and gathered information about personal characteristics, education and experience, job expectations, employment context information (such as quality of other job offers), and job characteristics. The second survey was completed 30 days after hire and gathered information about job characteristics (such as hours worked and salary), work-related characteristics (organizational commitment and job satisfaction), supervisor characteristics, employment context, training needs, and open-ended information about the job and how it could be improved. Two supplementary surveys were completed at the time of the second survey. One was the Leader Behavior Description Questionnaire (College of Administrative Science, 1957), and the other was the Organizational Socialization Survey (Jones, 1986). The third and fourth surveys gathered updated information about job characteristics (such as hours worked and salary), work-related characteristics (organizational commitment and job satisfaction), supervisor characteristics, employment context, training needs, and open-ended information about the job and how it could be improved. The third survey was administered after 6 months on the job and the fourth was administered after 12 months on the job. The final survey requested information from exiting employees about the person's leaving (e.g., was it voluntary? where did they go?), and about the good and bad aspects of the job. These surveys were administered in writing and were returned in sealed envelopes directly to the investigator. Supervisors completed a separate exit survey for direct support participants who left their position during the study; these questionnaires were completed either in writing or during a telephone interview.

The response rate for direct support workers ranged from 100% for the Time 1 survey to 28% for the staff exit questionnaire (see Table 9). Response rates were above 80% for all but Time 4 and the staff exit surveys.

Table 9. Return Rates for Direct Support Participant Surveys

Survey (when due)	# Expected	# Returned	% Returned
Time 1 (at hire)	174	174	100.00%
Time 2 (after 30 days)	158	138	87.34%
Organizational Socialization Survey (after 30 days)	142	126	88.73%
Leader Behavior Description Questionnaire (after 30 days)	158	138	87.34%
Time 3 (after 6 months)	109	90	82.57%
Time 4 (after 12 months)	72	54	75.00%
Staff exit (upon exit)	117	33	28.21%
Supervisor exit (upon exit)	117	116	99.15%

Table 10. Classification of Direct Support Workers

Months in Agency at Time 1[a]	Total # of Workers	Stayer			Leaver	Fired
		Stayed 12 Months	Promoted	Lateral Move	Left Voluntarily	Terminated
0-2	124	41	4	13	47	19
3-5	10	4	0	2	3	1
6-11	7	3	1	1	2	0
12+	20	13	0	4	3	0
Total N	161	61	5	20	55	20

[a] When starting in the studied home

The number of surveys expected varied depending on the number of direct support workers still employed at the time the survey was to have been completed. The Organizational Socialization Surveys were not included in the survey packets until 6 months after the project started, so some workers did not have the opportunity to complete that survey.

Of the 161 workers for whom current tenure was available, 124 were new to the agency at the time they were hired to work in the studied home (see Table 10). For the purpose of analysis, workers who stayed in the same home for 12 months, who were promoted within the agency, or who made a lateral move within the agency were considered stayers ($N = 58$). Workers who left the agency voluntarily were considered leavers ($N = 47$). Workers who were involuntarily terminated from employment were not included in comparisons of stayers and leavers. The 105 workers who were new to the agency and to the house who were not fired were included in the comparisons of stayers and leavers.

Instrumentation

The instruments used in this research were selected for one of three purposes. First, some instruments were selected because they provided information to describe the homes, residents, supervisors, or direct support workers studied. Second, many instruments were selected to measure specific constructs that were repeatedly found to be related to recruitment or retention outcomes. Chapter 3 provides an overview of the research that described these variables, and Table 5 summarizes many variables measured here. Finally, some instruments were selected because they describe recruitment, retention, or training outcomes for direct support workers or their supervisors. Published research instruments were used whenever possible to gather study information. Items not covered by an existing instrument were developed specifically for this study.

Facility Surveys

The facility surveys, which were administered to first-line supervisors, were designed to collect facility-level information about recruitment and retention outcomes in the homes in this study. The facility surveys asked about a wide range of facility, staff, and consumer characteristics and outcomes. This section highlights the measurement techniques and instruments used in the facility surveys.

Measures of Turnover

Crude Separation Rate. Turnover was measured using the crude separation rate defined by Price (1977) as follows:

$$\text{Crude Separation Rate} = \frac{\text{Number of members who left during the period}}{\text{Average number of members during the period}} \times 100$$

For this analysis, turnover during the previous 12 months was measured. Members are direct support workers who remained in any direct support position in the home during the 12 months. The average number of members in the period was estimated using the number of positions in a home at the time of the survey. For the remainder of this monograph, the terms "crude separation rate" and "turnover" are used interchangeably unless otherwise noted.

Average Tenure. Average tenure was defined as the total number of months all direct support workers in the home had been there divided by the total number of direct support workers in the home at the time of the analysis.

Ascension Rates. Ascension rates were defined as the number of new workers hired during the year divided by the average number of members in the year times 100.

Percentage of Leavers With Various Lengths of Tenure. The tenure of leavers was computed by identifying how many months each worker who left had worked in the home before leaving. The percentage who left before 6 months was the number who left before 6 months' tenure divided by the total number of leavers during the year. The percentage leaving in other periods were computed the same way.

Voluntariness and Avoidability of Leaving. Supervisor also provided information about workers who left to assess voluntariness, and avoidability of that leaving (Campion, 1991). Supervisor reports of voluntariness had an internal consistency rating of .90 among 548 supervisors, reports of avoidability had a rating of .90 among 545 supervisors, and reports of functionality had a rating of .88 among 549 supervisors.

Agency Management Practices
Response options for this question were drawn from a study in which respondents were asked to identify management practices that were important to controlling turnover (Pierson, 1993). Open-ended responses were then clustered into groups. For this study, the clusters were listed and respondents were asked to select the five most important management practices for addressing staffing issues.

Agency Management Problems
The response options for this question were drawn from Bruininks, et al. (1980). They reported the major problems for administrators in a national survey of residential facilities of all sizes. Additional problems were listed to incorporate issues identified by respondents in the pilot study.

Intensity of Supports Needed
A composite measure of intensity of supports needed was created using information collected in the facility surveys. Each person supported by a participating home was given a score ranging from 1 to 15 on this scale. The level of mental retardation was ranked on a five-point scale (1 = borderline or no

mental retardation, 5 = profound mental retardation). Challenging behavior was measured using two variables. A person received 2.5 points for the presence of a formal diagnosis of mental illness, and 2.5 points for having a specific planned intervention for challenging behavior. Finally, a person received one point for each of the following: if they needed assistance with walking, dressing, eating, or toileting, or if they did not communicate by talking. These scores were summed to create a single intensity of supports needed for each person. The average score for each home was then computed.

Other Questions
Information about facility characteristics was gathered using questions first developed for a national study of small group homes (Hill, et al., 1989). Data about population size and unemployment rates was obtained through review of U.S. Census population figures, and U.S. government local unemployment figures.

Direct Support Worker Surveys

Measures of Turnover
Staying or leaving was calculated based on whether the newly hired direct support workers remained in a direct support position in the home for 12 months after hire. New hires who were terminated involuntarily, transferred to another home, promoted, or left the agency voluntarily were specifically identified (see Jackofsky & Peters, 1983, for a discussion of the rationale behind counting those who transfer as leavers). Supervisor reports were used to identify leavers who were terminated involuntarily. Supervisors also indicated whether the workers who left their regular positions in the home continued to work "on-call" hours at the home after they left. Direct support workers who left were asked to complete Campion's (1991) scales for voluntariness and avoidability. Internal consistency ratings for voluntariness were

.92 for 307 employees, and for avoidability were .94 for 304 employees (Campion, 1991).

Organizational Commitment Questionnaire

Organizational commitment is "the relative strength of an individual's identification with and involvement in a particular organization," and is characterized by a strong belief in and acceptance of the organization's goals and values, a willingness to exert considerable effort on behalf of the organization, and a strong desire to maintain membership in the organization (Mowday, et al., 1982, p. 226). Although several instruments measure organizational commitment, the most commonly used scale is the Organizational Commitment Questionnaire (Mowday, et al., 1979). This 15-item scale has been normed on 2,563 employees in nine divergent occupations including psychiatric technicians working with people with mental retardation. Internal consistency ratings ranged from .82 to .93 with a median of .90. Test-retest reliabilities ranged from .53 to .75 over a 2- to 4-month period. Evidence of convergent, discriminant, and predictive validity were also presented by the authors. Other studies have confirmed high internal consistency ratings and comparatively better predictive validity for this scale than for other organizational commitment scales (e.g., Ferris & Aranya, 1983; Sullivan, 1982).

Minnesota Satisfaction Questionnaire

The Minnesota Satisfaction Questionnaire (MSQ) is one of three widely accepted measures of job satisfaction (Griffin & Bateman, 1986). According to the technical manual, the MSQ measures satisfaction with several different aspects of the work environment (Weiss, et al., 1967). The short form contains 20 items that measure satisfaction with the present job on a scale of 1 to 5. The MSQ yields three scale scores: intrinsic satisfaction, extrinsic satisfaction, and general satisfaction. Internal consistency ranged from .87 to .92 with a median of .90. Test-retest reliabilities were .89 over 1 week, and .70 over 1 year. Evidence supporting the validity of the MSQ and norms for 1,460 employees are presented in the manual. (This instrument is not included as an appendix because it is a copyrighted instrument.)

Job Expectations

The degree to which expectations about the job have been met has been considered an important variable in turnover research since Porter and Steers' (1973) review of the research. Wanous, et al. (1992), identified 18 studies that measured both job expectations and turnover. Although there have been several efforts to include this variable in turnover research, however, no single instrument has emerged as the dominant measure of job expectations. For this study the items from the Minnesota Satisfaction Questionnaire (Weiss, et al., 1967) were used to assess what the direct support workers expected from their job, and how important those things were to them. In addition, workers reported whether their job responsibilities and work conditions turned out to be what they expected, and whether the job overall met their original expectations. These questions were answered on a five-point likert scale with responses ranging from definitely yes to definitely no.

Staying or Leaving Index

While intent to stay or leave is often measured with a single item, an eight-item scale has been developed that provides a more stable index of intent (Bluedorn, 1982). The Staying or Leaving Index (SLI) contains four questions about the likelihood of still working for the organization over differing time spans, and four questions about the likelihood of quitting during four time spans. This index has an internal consistency ratio of .87 to .95 with a median of .91 for five samples of employees (Total $N = 741$).

Quality of Alternatives

The quality of alternative job opportunities was measured with a four-item scale that asks global questions about the employment outlook for an individual employee during the month before the survey (Rusbult, et al., 1988). Questions address the likelihood of getting a better job. Reliability and validity information were not available for this scale. A fifth item developed by these researchers, number of job offers in the past month, was included as a separate question.

Leader Behavior Descriptive Questionnaire

Leadership consideration of workers is one of the predictors of turnover identified in the Michaels and Spector (1982) turnover model (see Table 5). In this study, perception by the direct support workers of their supervisors was assessed using the Leader Behavior Descriptive Questionnaire (College of Administrative Science, 1957). Respondents rate the frequency that their supervisor engages in each behavior on a five-point likert scale. This instrument rates supervisors on initiating structure and consideration. Split-half reliability is .83 for the initiating structure scores, and .92 for consideration scores (Halpin, 1957). (This instrument is not included as an appendix because it is a copyrighted instrument.)

Prehire Organizational Knowledge

Prehire knowledge refers to how much a new worker knew about the job before he or she accepted it. It is measured in this study as a way of finding out how successful supervisors (and others) are at providing a realistic job preview to recruits who were actually hired. Prehire knowledge was measured using a six-item scale developed by Williams, et al. (1993). These items are measured on a five-point likert instrument. They ask how much people know about their job (1 = nothing, 5 = a great deal). The authors reported an internal consistency rating of .91 for this instrument.

Organizational Socialization

A socialization tactics scale developed by Jones (1986) was used to measure organizational socialization. This scale contained items measuring collective versus individual, formal versus informal, sequential versus variable, fixed versus variable, serial versus disjunctive, and investiture versus divestiture socialization tactics. The present analysis used items from this scale identified by Bachelder and Braddock (1994) as measuring informal co-worker support.

Satisfaction With Training

An eight-item scale developed by Larson and Hewitt (1995) was used to assess satisfaction with the training provided by the agency. The instrument uses a five-point likert scale. Internal consistency for this scale is .81.

Other Questions

Besides the instruments described here other items were developed using published items or scales when possible. Several job context variables were developed. For example, perceived job security was assessed using a single question from Arnold & Feldman (1982). Respondents provided a score from 1 (highly unlikely) to 7 (highly likely) for the question "How likely is it that you might be fired or laid off?" Job search activities were measured by asking the direct support workers which of several job search activities they have engaged in during the previous month (e.g., reading help wanted ads, submitting completed job applications, going on job interviews, networking with friends to identify possible job openings).

Most job characteristics variables were constructed with feedback from the instrument development team. The questions comparing pay with previous job and income needs were couched in the terms that Rice, et al. (1991), used for their perceived have-want discrepancy scale. A five-point scale was used for each of these one-item scales. The item about number of professional tasks was drawn from the scale used by Larson and Lakin (1992).

Procedures

Human Subjects Approval

The instruments and informed consent documents used for this research were submitted for approval to the Human Subjects Committee at the University of Minnesota and the State of Minnesota Institutional Review Board (for participating State Operated Community Services sites). Quarterly progress reports were provided to these agencies informing them of any changes or unexpected problems with the study.

Instrument Development

Academic professionals and stakeholders from the Department of Human Services staff, ARRM, and the SOCS administrative offices reviewed the instruments before their use. The proposed instruments were also completed and critiqued by five supervisors from community residential settings and four direct support workers. Once the instruments were reviewed, they were piloted in three study sites. Supervisors completed the facility Time 1 survey and invited one newly hired direct support worker to participate in the pilot project. This pilot test assessed not only the materials, but also the instructions and the procedures for delivering and returning the surveys, and for following participating houses. All of the surveys were modified slightly after the pilot study. The facility Time 2 survey was not developed until almost 1 year into the study. This allowed for changes that were clearly needed after checking responses to the first survey. The pilot study homes were included in the report of the results. Their responses were recorded on the revised form, with direct contact used to fill any gaps in the information.

Data Base Monitoring

A data base was developed to track receipt of letters of cooperation, supervisor consent forms, staff consent forms, and each survey for each facility and direct support worker participant. Monthly reports were used to monitor project status and to check for data entry errors.

Data Collection

Data collection began in December 1993 and was completed in December 1996. The study officially began in each home when the packet of surveys was delivered to a participating supervisor. From that point on, any new hires were to be invited to participate before their first shift at the home. To support the participating supervisors, monthly follow-up calls were made to the supervisors. Those calls:

- confirmed receipt of the survey packets,
- answered questions about carrying out of the study,
- prompted the supervisor to complete and return facility surveys,
- asked if any new direct support workers had been hired, and prompted supervisors to begin the study with them, asked if any participating direct support workers had left their positions and prompted supervisors to complete exit surveys, and
- notified supervisors of surveys due during the next month.

Additional calls were made to supervisors and participating direct support workers as needed to clarify responses on surveys returned and to gather data for questions that had been left blank.

Data Analysis Procedures

Facility Analysis

Descriptive statistics were used to describe facility characteristics, staffing patterns, staff characteristics, recruitment and retention characteristics, and resident characteristics.

Recruitment and retention outcomes were compared for homes funded by the ICF-MR program and those funded by the HCBS Waiver program and for homes at Time 1 and Time 2 using repeated measures analysis of variance. Descriptive statistics and qualitative analyses were used to summarize the strategies used by agencies to address recruitment and retention challenges. One-way ANOVA procedures were used to identify differences in turnover rates for agencies using various management strategies.

Multiple regression was used to identify the proportion of variability in annual turnover rates accounted for by a set of preselected variables (see Table 11). Two blocks of variables were force entered into the equation. The first block consisted of context and facility characteristics that were unlikely to be easily changed. The second block consisted of staffing patterns and strategies that individual agencies or homes could manipulate. The variables in these blocks were based on a match between the variables consistently associated with turnover in previous research, and the information collected in this study. The only exception was for the proportion of workers eligible for paid leave time. This study measured starting and top salary for workers and two forms of benefits—paid leave (e.g., sick, vacation, holiday, personal leave) and benefits (e.g., medical, dental, and other benefits). Either benefits or paid leave could have been included in the regression analysis. Paid leave was selected for inclusion because it is a more basic benefit than medical and other benefits. A qualitative analysis of open-ended responses was used to summarize issues and recommendations identified by supervisors. For each question, all responses were initially listed. The responses were subsequently each categorized by two researchers. The broad categories are reported in this monograph in order of how many workers mentioned a statement included in the category. A few examples of responses are provided for each category.

Table 11. Variables in Multiple Regression Analyses of Factors Associated With Turnover in Year 1 and Year 2

Contextual variables:

- Unemployment rate
- Percentage of state population in county of home

Facility characteristics:

- Average per diem
- Years open
- ICF-MR status

Resident characteristics:

- Intensity of need (level of MR, challenging behavior, adaptive behavior)

Staffing patterns:

- Starting wage
- Percentage eligible for paid leave
- Supervisor tenure in home
- Live-in staff

Individual-Level Analysis

The second set of analyses focuses on the surveys completed by newly hired direct support workers. Workers who stayed in the agency for 12 months were compared with those who voluntarily left within the first 12 months. Stayers and leavers were compared on demographic characteristics, educational background, recruitment experiences, job characteristics, conditions of employment, employment context, job attitudes, and socialization using descriptive statistics, one-way ANOVA, chi-square analyses, and repeated measures ANOVA with one within and one between subjects variables. Descriptive statistics were used to describe the survival rates of newly hired direct support workers. A discriminant analysis was used to identify the proportion of variability among new hires who did or did not stay for 12 months, accounted for by a set of preselected variables (See Table 12). Qualitative analyses were used to summarize worker comments regarding why they did or did not stay, the best and worst parts of the job, advice to potential new employees, and training needs for workers by noting each response made and categorizing those responses as noted above.

Table 12. Variables in a Discriminant Analysis of Stayers and Leavers

Personal characteristics:

- Age
- Months of experience

Context variables:

- Quality of alternative jobs

Job characteristics:

- Hours per week
- Hourly pay

Job outcomes:

- Organizational commitment
- General job satisfaction
- Stay/leave index score

Recruitment and socialization experiences:

- Internal recruitment source
- Met expectations
- Supervisor initiating structure score (LBDQ)

STUDY 1 RESULTS: FACILITY-LEVEL RECRUITMENT AND RETENTION ISSUES

The next two chapters describe the results of the two studies. They provide data to answer each of the research questions identified in chapter 2. Chapter 5 describes the findings of Study 1: the study of facilities and their supervisors (also called the facility-level analysis). Chapter 6 describes the findings of Study 2: the study of newly hired direct support workers. In both chapters, the quantitative findings are presented first followed by findings of open-ended questions of supervisors and direct support workers.

On-site supervisors in participating homes provided a range of information about the house and agency policies at the beginning of the study and again a year later. Most information in this chapter was gathered on the Time 1 facility survey. Selected variables from the Time 2 facility survey are also included. Each table notes the survey from which the data were drawn.

Characteristics of Participating Homes

As the first four research questions for the facility-level analysis focus on describing the characteristics of the homes, their supervisors, the direct support workers, and the conditions of employment for direct support workers in them, this chapter begins with a description of those characteristics. The 110 homes in this study supported an average of 4.5 individuals with mental retardation at an average cost per person per day of $169.96 (see Table 13). For ICFs-MR, the cost per day per person was the established per diem for the home. For HCBS Waiver homes the cost was calculated by summing the program costs for each person and the room and board rate (computed on a per day basis), and dividing by the number of people living in the home. Differences in cost per day by license type and by survey are provided later

Table 13. Context Characteristics (Time 1)

Characteristic	Mean	SD
State population living in county where home is located	8%	.09
Unemployment rate in country	3%	.01
Number of people in home	4.5	1.3
Daily cost per person	$169.96	$54.45
Year agency opened	1965.3	32.6
Number of sites in Minnesota	20.3	25.5
Year this site opened	1989.7	4.8
Direct support workers in union*	17%	.37

$N = 110$ homes except where noted, * $N = 109$

in this section. On average, the agency operating the home opened in 1965, with the typical home opening in mid-1989. Seventeen percent of the homes (all but one of which were state-operated homes) were unionized.

About two thirds of the homes (61%) were HCBS Waiver funded with the rest (39%) ICF-MR funded (see Table 14). Eighteen homes (16%) were state-operated, while the rest were fairly evenly divided between private profit (40%) and private nonprofit (44%) operation. Just over half the homes (52%) were located in Minnesota's Minneapolis/St. Paul metropolitan area with the next largest proportion (22%) in the Southeastern part of Minnesota.

For the purpose of comparison, the overall population of persons with mental retardation or related conditions in group or foster home settings in Minnesota in 1996 was 6,512 with 4,106 (63%) of those people in HCBS Waiver homes (Prouty & Lakin, 1997). The average daily cost per person in the ICF-MR program was $131.65, and the average daily cost for persons in the HCBS Waiver program was $108.75 (not including room and board) (Prouty & Lakin, 1997). In Minnesota, 91% of all congregate care residential settings had one to six residents (Prouty & Lakin, 1997). The homes in this study were similar to the statewide population in terms of the proportion of homes that were HCBS Waiver funded (61% vs. 63%). The cost for their care was above the statewide average. Several factors account for this difference including (a) about 18% of Minnesota's total HCBS Waiver recipients live in their family home at a cost substantially lower than for those living in out-of-home residential settings, thus lowering the overall average expenditure for Minnesota HCBS Waiver recipients, and (b) the homes in the study tended to be somewhat newer and supported people who were generally more impaired than Minnesota's overall community residential services recipients. The homes in this study all had six or fewer residents, like 91% of all congregate care residential settings in the state.

Table 14. Agency and Facility Characteristics (Time 1)

Characteristic	% of Homes
ICF-MR Certified	39%
HCBS Waiver	61%
Type of agency	
Public	16%
Private profit	40%
Private nonprofit	44%
Region of MN	
Metro	52%
Southeast	22%
Central	9%
Southwest	8%
Northeast	4%
Northwest	3%
West Central	2%

N = 110 homes

Characteristics of Residents

The facility survey requested information about each person living in the home. The average person supported was 41.5 years old (see Table 15) with just under half (47%) women. Of the people supported, 55% moved from one of Minnesota's Regional Treatment Centers (state institutions) to the home. Nearly two thirds of the residents had severe (26%) or profound (38%) mental retardation. Other common conditions included epilepsy (32%), brain or neurological damage (29%), a formal diagnosis of mental illness (26%), and blindness or uncorrected vision impairments (18%). Just over half of all residents had a specific planned intervention for challenging behavior (53%). Over half of all residents could walk without

Table 15. Resident Characteristics (Time 1)

Characteristic	Mean	SD
Number of residents	4.5	1.3
Average age	41.5	10.5
Female	47%	.34
Year moved to home	1990.7	3.1
Came from Regional Treatment Center	55%	.42
No mental retardation	2%	.06
Mild mental retardation	16%	.29
Moderate mental retardation	18%	.26
Severe mental retardation	26%	.31
Profound mental retardation	38%	.39
With current epilepsy or seizure disorder	32%	.26
With brain or neurological damage	29%	.37
With formal diagnosis of mental illness	26%	.32
Blind or have uncorrected vision impairments	18%	.23
With cerebral palsy	15%	.20
With autism	8%	.20
Deaf or have uncorrected hearing impairments	7%	.14
With specific planned intervention for challenging behavior	53%	.36
Walk without assistance	66%	.37
Eat without assistance	65%	.38
Communicate by talking	58%	.38
Independent in toileting (less than 1 daytime accident per month)	53%	.38
Dress without assistance	48%	.39

$N = 110$ homes

assistance (66%), eat without assistance (65%), communicate by talking (58%), and use the toilet independently with fewer than one daytime accident per month (53%). Just under half of all residents could dress without assistance (48%).

Supervisor Characteristics, Tasks, and Knowledge

First-line supervisors who participated in this study were overwhelmingly female (84%) (see Table 16). They averaged 34 years

Table 16.
Supervisor Characteristics

Characteristic	Mean	SD
Female	84%	.37
Mean age	33.6	9.2
Years in DD	9.3	5.5
Months in home	28.7	28.1
Years of school	15.8	1.5
Turnover (house level)	27.0%	–

$N = 110$ supervisors

old, and had 9 years of experience working with people who have developmental disabilities. The average supervisor had been in the home over 2 years (29 months), and had completed a bachelor's degree education (16 years of schooling). In the facilities surveyed, the turnover rate for supervisors was 27.0% over a 12-month period. That is, one of four supervisors left the home they were supervising for one reason or another (e.g., quit, transfer to another home, promotion, termination) during the year.

The average supervisor worked 34 hours per week at the sampled home including 11 hours doing direct care work and 22 hours doing supervisory tasks (see Table 17). The typical supervisor was responsible for supervising 10 direct support workers and 2.4 sites.

The most common supervisory responsibilities associated with recruitment and retention included providing house orientation (94%), providing ongoing training to workers (92%), interviewing applicants (87%), and hiring new employees (83%) (see Table 18). More than half of the supervisors were responsible for other staffing functions such as firing employees, responding to inquiries, screening applicants, providing agency orientation, and advertising job openings.

Supervisors indicated their level of knowledge about a wide range of training topics in five categories. Supervisors reported knowing the most about ensuring quality and integration of services (supervising provision of individual interventions and coordinating services across agencies), developing and maintaining operational systems (maintaining a safe and clean environment), and ensuring standards of

Table 17. Supervisor Tasks

Task	Mean	SD	# of Homes
Supervisor tasks (Time 2)			
Total hours worked at home per week	34.0	14.7	74
Hours of direct care at this home per week	10.9	11.2	90
Hours of supervisory tasks at this home per week	21.6	11.5	96
Number of people supervised (Time 2)			
DSWs	10.1	5.6	80
Supervisors	0.5	0.9	80
Professional support staff	0.5	0.8	80
Other support staff	0.2	0.4	80
Number of sites supervised	2.4	3.3	96

Table 18. Recruitment and Retention Tasks for Supervisors

Task	% of Homes
Performance reviews	97%
Providing house orientation	94%
Providing ongoing training	92%
Interviewing applicants	87%
Hiring new employees	83%
Firing employees	78%
Responding to inquiries	73%
Screening applicants	66%
Providing agency orientation	65%
Advertising job openings	55%
Average # tasks per supervisor	8.0

$N = 110$ homes

compliance (reviewing and monitoring program activities for standards compliance) (see Table 19). They reported knowing least about providing leadership and management of staff (conducting performance reviews, supervising and training staff) and developing and maintaining community relations (establishing and maintaining relationships with families, friends, and community members). In general they felt they were most knowledgeable about topics related to maintaining compliance to rules and regulations, and least about categories related to providing good leadership and management of community-oriented residential supports. The average rating in each of the five categories was above 3.0 indicating that, on average, the supervisors felt they "knew a lot" about the topics investigated.

Characteristics of Direct Support Workers

Most direct support workers in the homes studied were female (78%). Their average age was 32 years. Direct support workers in these homes worked an average of 28 hours per week (see Table 20). A few homes used night staff permitted to sleep (18%), but in most homes at least one staff member was required to remain awake throughout the night. The majority (81%) of newly hired direct support workers were required to complete a probationary period which on average lasted 4.1 months.

Staffing patterns varied depending on the time of day. The number of workers ranged from 1.35 on duty at 2:00 A.M. to 2.35

Table 19. Supervisor Knowledge of Training Topics (Time 2)

Topic Category	Mean	SD
Ensuring quality and integration of services	3.38	0.43
Developing and maintaining operational systems	3.32	0.48
Ensuring standards of compliance	3.23	0.59
Providing leadership and management of staff	3.08	0.42
Developing and maintaining community relations	3.01	0.56

$N = 80$ supervisors
4 = I know the topic well enough to provide advanced training to other supervisors.
3 = I know a lot about the topic but could benefit from advanced training.
2 = I know about the topic but could benefit from basic training.
1 = I know little and could benefit from a basic introduction and comprehensive training.

Table 20. Direct Support Worker Characteristics (Time 1)

Characteristics	Mean % of Homes	SD
Average age of DSWs	31.9	(5.9)
Female	76%	(0.19)
Average hours per week at the house per worker	27.8	(5.5)
Homes using asleep night staff	18%	
Homes using a probationary period	81%	
Number of months in probationary period*	4.1	(1.8)

$N = 110$ homes except where noted, * $N = 96$ homes

Table 21. Direct Support Worker Staffing Patterns (Time 1)

Characteristics	Mean % of Homes	SD
Number of staff on duty		
7:30 A.M. weekdays	1.99	0.82
3:00 P.M. weekdays	2.15	0.81
7:30 P.M. weekdays	2.29	0.76
2:00 A.M. weekdays	1.35	0.48
7:30 A.M. weekends	1.82	0.76
3:00 P.M. weekends	2.35	0.77
7:30 P.M. weekends	2.15	0.72
2:00 A.M. weekends	1.35	0.48
Staff per resident 3:00 P.M. weekdays	0.48	0.16
Number and type of staff		
DSW regular shifts	9.47	3.63
DSW "on-call"	2.52	3.09
Direct supervisors	2.61	2.82
Total staff per resident	2.12	0.64
FTE DSW per resident	1.44	0.41
Homes using live-in staff	18%	

$N = 110$ homes

on duty on weekend afternoons (see Table 21). In the afternoon when everyone was home, there was an average of one direct support worker for every two residents. The total staff complement for these small homes averaged 2.12 workers per resident with the number of full-time equivalent (FTE) workers averaging 1.44 per resident. A total of 18% of the homes used live-in staff members for at least part of their staff complement. The typical home had 9.5 direct support workers with regularly scheduled shifts, 2.5 direct support workers who did not work regularly scheduled hours but only "on-call" shifts, and 2.6 supervisors, who as noted devoted about one third of their work time to direct support of residents.

Virtually all of the homes expected direct support workers to prepare meals (100%), provide resident transportation (99%), do laundry (98%), and clean the home (97%) (see Table 22). Some homes also required direct support workers to do gardening, shoveling or mowing, or building maintenance or repair.

In most homes, at least some direct

Table 22. Basic Care-Giving Tasks Performed by Direct Support Workers

Tasks	Mean (SD)/ % of Homes
Prepare meals	100%
Provide resident transportation	99%
Laundry	98%
Cleaning	97%
Gardening and lawn maintenance	56%
Building maintenance or repair	32%
Total number of basic care tasks	4.8 (0.9)

$N = 110$ homes

Table 23. Professional Tasks Performed by Direct Support Workers

Tasks	Mean (SD)/ % of Homes
Attend program planning meetings	83%
Set up program plans or meetings	60%
Supervise other staff or schedule shifts	56%
Write program plans	55%
Hire replacements	18%
Total number of professional tasks	2.7 (1.6)

$N = 110$ homes

Table 24. Professional Support Staff On-Site

Support Staff	Mean (SD)/ % of Homes
Nurse (RN or LPN)	89%
Nutritionist or dietician	51%
Behavior analyst or consultant	36%
Psychologist	32%
Occupational therapist	31%
Psychiatrist	24%
Physical therapist	20%
Speech, language, or communication therapist	18%
Social worker (noncounty)	16%
Advocate	12%
Recreation therapist	4%
Total number of professional supports provided	3.5 (2.3)

$N = 110$ homes

support workers were expected to participate in program planning meetings (83%), set up program planning meetings (60%), supervise other staff members (56%), or write program plans (55%) (see Table 23). Only a few homes (18%) involved direct support workers in hiring replacement workers.

The availability of professional and other support staff members varied across homes (see Table 24). While most homes had a nurse (89%) who provided services on-site and 51% had on-site nutritionists/dieticians, one third or fewer had on-site behavioral analysts or behavioral consultants, psychologists, occupational therapists, psychiatrists, or other therapists.

The most commonly available nonprofessional support was a maintenance or repair person (available in 82% of the homes) (see Table 25). More than half of the homes had support staff members to do gardening or lawn maintenance, while only a few homes had drivers, cleaning persons, or cooks.

Table 25. Support Staff On-Site

Support Staff	Mean (SD)/ % of Homes
Maintenance or repair person	82%
Gardener or lawn maintenance	58%
Driver	14%
Cleaning person	10%
Cook	3%
Laundry	0%
Total number of other support staff	1.7 (0.9)

$N = 110$ homes

Wages, Benefits, and Staff Tenure

The average minimum beginning wage was $7.07 per hour for awake staff and $5.39 per hour for asleep night staff members (see Table 26). The average highest wage was $9.27 per hour for awake staff while the average highest wage for asleep night staff was $6.43 per hour. On average, direct support workers had to work 35 hours per week to be considered full time, 18.5 hours

Table 26. Wages and Eligibility for Benefits

Characteristics	Mean	SD
Awake beginning wage	$7.07	$1.40
Awake maximum wage	$9.27	$2.48
Asleep beginning wage	$5.39	$1.55
Asleep maximum wage	$6.43	$2.76
Number of hours considered full time	35.2	4.5
DSWs in the home who are full time	43%	.20
Hours per week to be eligible for paid leave	18.5	14.0
DSWs in the home who are eligible for paid leave	72%	.31
Hours per week to be eligible for benefits	27.6	8.2
DSWs in the home who are eligible for benefits	59%	.27

$N = 110$ homes

per week to be eligible for paid leave time (holidays, vacation, sick, personal leave), and 27.6 hours per week to be eligible for benefits (health, dental, retirement, other). Of all the workers, 43% were considered full time by these standards, while 71% were eligible for paid leave, and 59% were eligible for benefits.

Factors in Establishing Beginning, Differential, and Increased Wages

Homes varied in the factors they considered when establishing beginning, differential, and increased wages for workers (see Table 27). The most common criteria for setting initial wages for direct support workers included job title (56% of the homes), experience in the field (48%), and educational background (43%).

Most homes reported offering overtime pay for working more than 40 hours in 1 week (85%). Most also offered differential pay for working holiday shifts (78%) (see Table 28). Fewer than one third of the homes offered differential pay for overnight shifts (31%), evening hours (15%), weekend hours (13%), or working full time (13%).

Factors considered when determining the amount of raises also varied (see Table 29). More than half of the homes considered performance (75%), number of months worked (68%), or promotion to a higher level direct support position (57%). Fewer homes considered increased responsibilities (43%), increased hours (15%), or changes in union contracts (14%) as factors in pay increases.

The number of 8-hour days of paid leave (including holidays) available after 1 year averaged 25.8 for workers who worked 40 hours per week, and 8.5 (68 hours) for workers who worked 20 hours per week (see Table 30). Each agency used a different combination of sick, vacation, holiday, paid leave time and other categories to reach the total number of days available. Some agencies provided paid leave as a chunk of hours to be used at the discretion of the employee rather than providing a specific

Table 27. Factors Influencing Starting Wages

Factors	% of Homes
Job title	56%
Experience in the field	48%
Other	45%
Educational background	43%
Number of hours per week	16%

$N = 110$ homes

Table 28. Factors Influencing Pay Differentials

Factors	% of Homes
More than 40 hours per week	85%
Holidays	78%
Overnight shifts	31%
Other	27%
Evening hours	15%
Weekend hours	13%
Full-time status	13%

$N = 110$ homes

Table 29. Factors Influencing Wage Increases

Factors	% of Homes
Performance review	75%
Number of months worked	68%
Promotion as DSW	57%
Increased responsibilities	43%
Increase in hours	15%
Other	15%
Changes in union contract	14%

$N = 110$ homes

Table 30. Direct Support Worker Paid Leave

Facility Characteristics	Mean	SD	# of Homes
FT paid leave days after 1 year			
Sick	5.9	5.5	105
Vacation	7.1	5.9	106
Holiday	5.8	4.5	106
Paid leave	4.7	7.6	105
Other	5.1	9.6	70
Total	25.8	8.6	110
PT (50%FTE) paid leave days after 1 year			
Sick	2.2	3.0	105
Vacation	2.6	3.0	106
Holiday	1.9	3.4	105
Paid leave	1.2	5.7	106
Other	1.3	3.8	70
Total	8.5	8.0	110

Note: A day is 8 hours for this table. A part-time person working 4 hours per shift would have two shifts off when given 8 hours of leave.

number of sick, vacation, or holiday days off. Some agencies provided paid leave to part-time workers on a prorated basis if the worker met a minimum threshold of hours per week.

Most full-time direct support workers could obtain health insurance for themselves (see Table 31). The agency paid 100% of the cost of health insurance for full-time workers in 36% of the agencies, some but not all of the cost in 61% of the agencies, and offered insurance the worker could purchase by paying full cost in 2% of the agencies. The most common benefit paid for entirely by the employer was life insurance (69% of all agencies), followed by retirement in addition to Social Security (46%), health insurance for the worker (36%), and other benefits such as mileage or food (29%). Direct support workers who averaged 20 hours per week could access health and dental insurance for themselves and their families in fewer than half the homes. The most common benefits for 20-hour-per-week workers included retirement (34% of all agencies), life insurance (31%), and other benefits (11%). The most common arrangement for 20-hour-per-week workers was to have the employer pay part of the cost for health insurance for the worker (40% of all homes), the worker's dependents (38%), and dental insurance for the worker (37%) and the worker's dependents (35%).

Table 31. Direct Support Worker Benefits (Time 1)

Benefits at Time 1	# of Homes	Employer Contribution			
		100%	1% to 99%	Offered 0%	Not Offered
FT benefits (for 100% FTE employee)					
Health insurance (self)	110	36%	61%	2%	2%
Health insurance (dependents)	110	7%	60%	29%	4%
Dental plan (self)	110	25%	53%	5%	18%
Dental plan (dependents)	110	7%	47%	24%	22%
Life insurance (self)	110	69%	14%	6%	11%
Retirement (other than Social Security)	110	46%	25%	7%	22%
Child care	110	0%	2%	21%	77%
Tuition	108	4%	28%	0%	68%
Other	58	29%	24%	5%	41%
Total number of benefits	110	1.44	2.35	.65	.56
PT benefits (for 50% FTE employee)					
Health insurance (self)	110	4%	40%	2%	55%
Health insurance (dependents)	110	1%	38%	6%	55%
Dental plan (self)	110	2%	37%	2%	59%
Dental plan (dependents)	110	0%	35%	6%	59%
Life Insurance (self)	109	31%	6%	6%	57%
Retirement (other than Social Security)	110	34%	20%	6%	41%
Child care	110	0%	1%	15%	85%
Tuition	108	2%	17%	0%	82%
Other	57	11%	25%	5%	60%
Total number of benefits	110	.37	1.56	.22	2.84

Note: Totals may not equal 100% due to rounding.

Table 32. Agency Management Practices and Problems (Time 1)

Practices and Problems	% of Homes
Difficulty finding qualified staff	57%
Staff turnover	44%
Staff motivation	37%
Funding mechanism problems (e.g., late checks, county control)	32%
Maintenance, physical plant, capital expenditures	30%
Wage and hour considerations	29%
Government regulations	24%
Problems with residents	24%
Staff training and development	23%
Staffing patterns and work conditions	22%
Inadequate funds	20%
Lack of community support services	20%
Lack of coordination between provider agencies	15%
Community attitudes toward residents	15%
Start-up money and costs	15%
Lack of program implementation	15%
Need for transportation services	14%
Problems with family members	11%
Certification and licensing	11%
Developing individualized program plans	9%
Lack of advocacy services	7%
Workmen's compensation	7%
Lack of comprehensive state planning	6%
Lack of alternative community residential placements	5%
Unions/labor relations	5%
Lack of follow-along services	5%
Quality assurance	4%
Relationship with board of directors	4%
Admissions policies	3%
Insurance problems	1%
Difficulty maintaining sufficient average daily resident population	1%

$N = 110$ homes

Table 33. Limitations of New Hires (Time 1)

Limitations	Mean (SD)/ % of Homes
Lack of DD experience	60%
Lack of experience with job responsibilities	39%
Lack of specific training	38%
Lack of maturity	32%
Lack basic communication skills	25%
Other	15%
No limitations	12%
Number of limitations reported per supervisor	2.1 (1.3)

$N = 110$ homes

Recruitment and Retention Outcomes

Agency Management Practices and Problems

Supervisors indicated whether they experienced difficulties with each of 37 issues that had previously been identified as problems for community residential facilities (Bruininks, et al., 1980). The two most common difficulties repeated by supervisors were finding qualified staff members (57% of all homes) and staff turnover (44%). Staff motivation was also a commonly reported difficulty (37%) (see Table 32). Funding mechanism problems and maintenance, physical plant, and capital expenditure issues were reported by more than 30% of the supervisors.

When asked about specific recruitment problems, most supervisors reported that new hires were limited because of a lack of experience supporting people with developmental disabilities (DD) (60% of homes)

(see Table 33). Other limitations of new hires included lack of experience with job responsibilities (39% of homes), lack of specific training (38%), and a general lack of maturity (32%).

Differential Outcomes for ICF-MR Versus HCBS Waiver Homes at Time 1 and Time 2

A repeated measures analysis of variance with one within (time) and one between (type of facility) factors was used to measure how recruitment and retention outcomes varied over time and across facility type. Tables 34 and 35 show the means for each type at each time on each variable, overall means (and standard deviations) at Time 1 and Time 2 for each variable, and the results of each component of the repeated measures analysis for each variable.

There were no statistically significant differences between ICF-MR and HCBS Waiver homes or between measurements at Time 1 and Time 2 in the percentage of supervisors who reported difficulties finding new direct support workers, the proportion of applicants offered a position, satisfaction with the most recent new hire, the number of direct support workers promoted in the last year, and the number of direct support workers moving from part-time to full-time positions in the last year. The differences in cost per person per day were also not statistically significant in this study. Overall 64% of supervisors reported having problems finding new direct support workers at Time 1, and 68% reported difficulties at Time 2. Supervisors hired more than half of all applicants at Time 1 (53%) and at Time 2 (56%). Supervisors were moderately satisfied with the new hires at Time 1 (2.2) and at Time 2 (2.3). Supervisors reported promoting 6 direct support workers for every 100 positions in the homes, and reported moving 11 direct support workers for every 100 positions from part-time positions to full-time positions in the previous year. Between

Table 34. Recruitment and Retention Difficulties in ICF-MR and HCBS Homes: Group Means and Repeated Measures ANOVA Results

Outcome	Time 1		Time 2		Total		F	F	F
	ICF-MR N=38	HCBS Waiver N=56	ICF-MR N=38	HCBS Waiver N=56	Time 1 Mean (SD) N=94	Time 2 Mean (SD) N=94	Time 1 vs. Time 2	ICF-MR vs. Waiver	Interaction
Cost per person per day	$187.26	$155.15	$183.10	$172.19	$168.31 (54.54)	$176.60 (77.34)	0.66	3.41	1.82
Homes reporting problems finding new DSWs	61%	66%	74%	64%	64% (.48)	68% (.47)	1.11	0.09	1.89
Applicants offered job	42%	59%	52%	58%	53% (.59)	56% (.38)	0.61	1.45	0.84
Satisfaction with new hire	2.3	2.2	2.4	2.2	2.2 (1.2)	2.3 (1.2)	0.08	0.72	0.02
Difficulty caused by turnover	2.8	2.8	2.6	2.6	2.8 (.92)	2.6 (.98)	4.19*	0.00	0.05
DSWs promoted	4%	8%	5%	6%	6% (.11)	6% (.11)	0.01	0.00	0.05
DSWs moving from PT to FT	8%	12%	8%	12%	11% (.14)	11% (.12)	0.01	2.72	0.00

*$p < .05$
Difficulty caused by turnover (1 = very much, 4 = very little or none)
Satisfaction with new hire (1 = very satisfied, 6 = very dissatisfied)

Table 35. Recruitment and Retention Outcomes for ICF-MR and HCBS Homes: Repeated Measures ANOVA

Outcome	Time 1 ICF-MR N=38	Time 1 HCBS Waiver N=56	Time 2 ICF-MR N=38	Time 2 HCBS Waiver N=56	Total Time 1 Mean (SD) N=94	Total Time 2 Mean (SD) N=94	F Time 1 vs. Time 2	F ICF-MR vs. Waiver	F Interaction
Average tenure (months)	23.6	17.0	31.7	22.3	19.6 (13.3)	26.1 (16.4)	27.5***	6.61*	1.22
DSWs with more than 12 months' tenure	72%	59%	90%	85%	65% (.23)	87% (.15)	50.44***	6.05*	2.02
Crude separation rate	45%	47%	45%	51%	46% (.37)	48% (.42)	0.29	0.25	0.34
Ascension rate			19%	37%		30% (.34)		6.39*	
DSWs who left before 6 months' tenure	37%	50%	30%	41%	45% (.36)	36% (.34)	2.25	4.12*	0.06
DSWs who left 6 - 12 months' tenure	29%	19%	19%	26%	23% (.27)	23% (.29)	0.14	0.14	2.81
DSWs who left after 12 months' tenure	35%	31%	51%	34%	32% (.36)	41% (.36)	3.56	2.73	1.63

* p < .05, *** p < .001

Time 1 and Time 2, the difficulty caused by turnover increased significantly, $F(1,94) = 4.19, p < .05$ from 2.8 to 2.6 (1 = very much, 4 = very little). There were no differences between ICF-MR homes and HCBS Waiver homes in the difficulty caused by turnover. Considering that the greatest challenge facing these supervisors is recruitment (see Table 32), increasing problems with recruitment could explain the increase in the difficulties caused by turnover in these homes.

The crude separation rates were 46% at Time 1 and 48% at Time 2. The rates did not differ by time or by type of home. There were, however, significant differences in another measure of turnover. Specifically, a one-way analysis of variance (ANOVA) showed significant differences between ICF-MR and HCBS Waiver homes at Time 2 in the accession rate, $F(1,93) = 6.39, p < .05$. ICF-MR homes hired 19.3 new workers for every 100 positions while HCBS Waiver homes hired 36.9 new workers for every 100 direct support positions in the previous year. HCBS Waiver funded homes hired workers significantly more often than ICF-MR funded homes.

Differences were observed in overall tenure of workers in the homes, and in tenure of leavers. The average tenure of all workers in the homes was significantly higher for ICF-MR homes (23.6 months at Time 1 and 31.7 months at Time 2) than for HCBS Waiver homes (17.0 months at Time 1 and 22.3 months at Time 2), $F(1,76) = 6.61$, $p < .05$. Overall tenure also increased significantly overall between Time 1 and Time 2 (from 19.6 months to 26.1 months) $F(1,76) = 27.5, p < .001$. Changes in the proportion of direct support workers in each home with more than 12 months' tenure mirrored changes in the average tenure of workers in the home. A significantly higher proportion of ICF-MR workers (72% at Time 1 and 90% at Time 2) had more than 12 months' tenure compared with HCBS Waiver workers (59% at Time 1 and 85% at Time 2),

$F(1,62) = 6.06, p < .05$. As with average tenure, the proportion of workers with 12 months tenure in the home also increased significantly between Time 1 and Time 2 (from 65% to 87%), $F(1,62) = 50.44, p < .001$. Finally, there was a significant difference in the proportion of leavers who had been in the home less than 6 months before they quit. Specifically, new workers in ICF-MR homes were less likely to leave within the first 6 months (37% at Time 1 and 30% at Time 2) than were new workers in HCBS Waiver homes (50% at Time 1 and 41% at Time 2), $F(1,72) = 4.12, p < .05$.

To understand the differences in recruitment and retention outcomes, it is helpful to know that ICF-MR homes in this study opened, on average, in 1988 ($SD = 5.9$ years) while HCBS Waiver homes opened in 1991 ($SD = 3.5$ years). In a one-way analysis of variance this difference is statistically significant, $F(1,108) = 15.25, p < .001$) This information along with the changes observed between Time 1 and Time 2 in tenure of workers suggests that retention outcomes, particularly those measuring tenure, improve as a home has been open longer.

Factors Associated With Differences in Retention Outcomes

While the rate at which workers left the organization did not differ over time nor was it based on the type of facility, several other factors were associated with facility-level turnover rates. Table 36 shows the correlation between variables measured at Time 1 (looking back over the previous year), and turnover, average tenure, and the proportion of workers with more than 12 months' tenure at Time 1 and at Time 2. Variables with significant correlations with turnover (i.e., crude separation rate) at Time 1 included the population of the county in which the home was located ($r = .20, p < .05$), supervisor tenure in the home ($r = -.23, p < .05$), the proportion of direct support workers eligible for paid leave ($r = -.34, p < .01$), and the

Table 36. Correlations with Facility-Level Retention Outcomes

Variable @ Time 1	Turnover @ Time 1	Turnover @ Time 2	Tenure @ Time 1	Tenure @ Time 2	% 12+ Months' Tenure @ Time 1	%12+ Months' Tenure @ Time 2
	(# of Homes)	(# of Homes)	(# of Homes)	(# of Homes)	(# of Homes)	(# of Homes)
Unemployment rate	-.18 (110)	.02 (96)	.11 (109)	.26* (79)	.23* (90)	.23* (78)
% of state population in county where home is located	.20* (110)	.07 (96)	-.17 (109)	-.08 (79)	-.22* (90)	-.07 (78)
Average per diem	.13 (109)	.04 (95)	-.19 (108)	-.22* (78)	.02 (89)	.24* (77)
Years home open	.00 (110)	.01 (96)	.48** (109)	.58** (79)	.14 (90)	.00 (78)
ICF-MR status	-.04 (110)	-.07 (96)	.25** (109)	.27* (79)	.26* (90)	.14 (78)
Starting pay	-.13 (110)	-.28** (96)	.02 (109)	-.00 (79)	.22* (90)	.20 (78)
Use live-in workers	-.05 (110)	.08 (96)	-.18 (109)	-.24* (79)	-.13 (90)	-.21 (78)
Resident case mix	.19 (109)	.06 (95)	-.16 (108)	-.14 (78)	-.10 (89)	.28* (77)
Supervisor tenure in home	-.23* (110)	-.24* (96)	.49** (109)	.65** (79)	.32** (90)	-.02 (78)
% DSW eligible for paid leave	-.34** (92)	-.13 (92)	.09 (91)	.05 (77)	.42** (75)	.26* (76)
% DSW eligible for benefits	-.10 (92)	-.07 (92)	.01 (91)	.04 (77)	.24* (75)	.53** (76)
# DSW promoted in year	.34** (110)	.13 (96)	-.13 (109)	-.09 (79)	-.21* (90)	.28* (78)

$* p < .05, ** p < .01$

number of direct support workers promoted in the previous year ($r = .34, p < .01$). Turnover at Time 2 was significantly correlated with starting pay for direct support workers at Time 1 ($r = -.28, p < .01$), and supervisor tenure in the home at Time 1 ($r = -.24, p < .05$).

As reported, the average tenure of workers at Time 1 was significantly correlated with years the home was open and with ICF-MR status. In addition, average tenure at Time 1 was significantly correlated with supervisor tenure at Time 1 ($r = .49, p < .01$). Average tenure of workers at Time 2 was significantly correlated with years the home was open, ICF-MR status, and supervisor tenure in the home at Time 1. In addition, average tenure at Time 2 was significantly correlated with the county unemployment rate at Time 1 ($r = .26, p < .05$), average cost per person per day at Time 1 ($r = -.22, p < .05$), whether live-in workers were used at the home ($r = -.24, p < .05$), and supervisor tenure in the home ($r = .65, p < .01$).

Finally, the proportion of workers in each home that had been in the home for more than 12 months was associated with several variables. For the proportion with more than 12 months' tenure at Time 1, significant correlations were reported for unemployment rate ($r = .23, p < .05$), the population of the county in which the home was located ($r = -.22, p < .05$), ICF-MR status ($r = .26, p < .05$), supervisor tenure in the home ($r = .32, p < .01$), the proportion of direct support workers eligible for paid leave ($r = .42, p < .01$), the proportion of direct support workers eligible for benefits ($r = .24, p < .05$), and the number of direct support workers promoted in the previous year ($r = -.21, p < .05$). The proportion of workers with more than 12 months' tenure at Time 2 was significantly correlated with the unemployment rate at Time 1 ($r = .23, p < .05$), the average cost per resident per day at Time 1 ($r = .24, p < .05$), the overall difficulty of care for residents (level of mental retardation, challenging behavior, adaptive behavior)

Table 37. Regression Results for Turnover at Time 1

Variable @ Time 1 (Final model)	Unstandardized Coefficients B	SE	Standardized Coefficient Beta	t
Constant	83.80	30.27		2.77**
Block 1				
Unemployment rate	-2.24	3.61	-.06	-.62
County population (% of state population)	29.97	43.10	.07	.69
Average per diem	0.14	0.09	.21	1.68
Years home open	1.47	0.94	.19	1.56
ICF-MR status	-4.56	8.16	-.06	-.56
Resident case mix	4.24	1.81	.27	2.35*
Block 2				
Starting pay	-8.49	3.23	-.30	-2.63**
Use live-in workers	1.24	10.02	.01	.12
Supervisor tenure in home	-0.30	0.14	-.24	-2.11*
% DSW eligible for paid leave	-0.39	0.13	-.31	-3.05**

* $p < .05$, ** $p < .01$
Full model $R^2 = .34$, Adjusted $R^2 = .26$, $F(10, 79) = 4.07, p < .001$
$N = 90$ homes

Table 38. Regression Results for Turnover at Time 2

Variable @ Time 1 (Final model)	Unstandardized Coefficients B	SE	Standardized Coefficient Beta	t
Constant	78.73	36.76		2.14*
Block 1				
Unemployment rate	2.92	4.39	.08	0.67
County population (% of state population)	64.00	52.33	.14	1.22
Average per diem	0.19	0.10	.25	1.80
Years home open	1.18	1.14	.14	1.03
ICF-MR status	-4.12	9.91	-.05	-0.42
Resident case mix	1.87	2.19	.11	0.85
Block 2				
Starting pay	-11.32	3.92	-.36	-2.89**
Use live-in workers	6.24	12.17	.06	0.51
Supervisor tenure in home	-0.33	0.17	-.24	-1.93
% DSW eligible for paid leave	-0.10	0.16	-.07	-0.66

$* p < .05, ** p < .01$
$R^2 = .21$, Adjusted $R^2 = .11$, $F(10, 79) = 2.08, p < .05$
N = 90 homes

$(r = .28, p < .05)$, the proportion of workers eligible for paid leave $(r = .26, p < .05)$, the proportion of workers eligible for benefits $(r = .53, p < .01)$, and the number of direct support workers promoted at Time 1 $(r = .28, p < .05)$. All of the variables identified at Time 1 as potentially related to retention outcomes were significantly correlated with at least one outcome.

Two blocks of variables were tested to determine their contribution to explaining the variability in turnover rates. The first block included context, facility, and resident characteristics that could affect turnover. The second block included staffing patterns and strategies. A multiple regression analysis accounted for 34% of the variability (26% adjusted) in

Table 39. Use of Temporary Agency Services (Time 2)

Temporary Service	Mean (SD)/ % of Homes	# of Homes
Homes using temporary agency services	18%	96
Satisfaction with temporary agency services	2.2 (0.8)	17
Number of shifts used in last month	2.7 (5.8)	29

Satisfaction (1 = very satisfied, 5 = very dissatisfied)

Table 40. Helpfulness of Various Recruitment Strategies (Time 2)

Strategies	Mean	SD	# of Homes (% using strategy)
Newspaper advertisements	2.20	0.61	86 (78%)
Recruitment by current or former employees	2.13	0.71	84 (76%)
Internal posting	1.98	0.73	84 (76%)
High school, technical college, or college placement office/job board	1.69	0.62	62 (56%)
Employment/referral agency	1.67	0.76	30 (27%)
TV or radio advertisements	1.00	0.0	4 (4%)
Other	2.33	0.52	6 (6%)

3 = Very helpful, 2 = Somewhat helpful, 1 = Not helpful
Effectiveness for Those Who Use the Strategy

Table 41. Recruitment Incentives for Current Workers Who Recruit New Workers (Time 2)

Incentive	% of Homes
Financial only	35%
Other only (e.g., paid time off)	4%
Both financial and other incentives used	3%
Incentives not used	59%

$N = 80$ homes

turnover rates at Time 1 using variables including unemployment rate, county population, average cost per resident, years home was open, ICF-MR status, resident case mix score, starting pay for direct support workers, whether live-in staff were used, the tenure of the supervisor in the home, and the percentage of direct support workers eligible for paid leave, $F(10, 89) = 4.07, p < .001$ (see Table 37). Unique contributions to explaining the variability in turnover rates at Time 1 were made by resident support needs, starting pay for direct support workers, supervisor tenure in

the home, and the proportion of direct support workers eligible for paid leave.

The same set of variables accounted for a statistically significant 21% (11% adjusted) of the variability in turnover rates at Time 2, $F(10, 79) = 2.08, p < .05$ (see Table 38). In the Time 2 equation, however, only starting pay at Time 1 made a unique contribution to explaining the variability of turnover rates.

Responses and Strategies Used to Address Recruitment and Retention Challenges

Responses to recruitment and retention challenges varied for the agencies in this study. Some agencies (18%) reported using temporary agencies to fill vacancies due to turnover (see Table 39). The 17 agencies that used temporary agencies reported an average satisfaction rating of 2.2 (somewhat satisfied) with the services. The average home used temporary workers to fill 2.7 shifts in a 1-month period.

Supervisors indicated how often they used several different recruitment strategies along with how effective they felt the strategy

Table 42. Realistic Job Preview Strategies Used by Supervisors

Use of RJPs	Mean (SD)/ % of Homes
Use realistic job previews	95%
Verbal descriptions	89%
Direct observation of people in the home	46%
Written information	35%
Audio or video information	3%
Other	2%
Number of RJP strategies used per home	1.8 (0.9)
DSWs who see job description before hire	51%(.50)

$N = 96$ homes

was (see Table 40). The most frequently used strategies to communicate about an existing opening were newspaper advertisements (used by 78% of the supervisors), recruitment by current or former employees (76%), and internal posting of openings (76%). These three strategies were also reported to be the most useful on a scale of 1 to 3 with 3 indicating very helpful and 1 indicating not helpful (2.2 for newspaper advertisements, 2.1 for recruitment by current or former employees, and 2.0 for internal postings). Job boards and employment or referral agencies were used less often and were reported to be less effective strategies for recruiting new workers.

Two strategies to address recruitment and retention problems identified in prior research as potentially helpful were specifically studied. One strategy involves providing incentives to current employees who recruit new staff members (used to increase inside recruiting). A total of 41% of the homes in this study used incentives to improve inside recruitment (see Table 41). Most homes (35%) provided financial incentives for recruiting new workers. A few homes provided other types of incentives, such as paid time off (4%) or offered both financial and other types of incentives (3%).

The other strategy was the use of realistic job previews (RJPs). The researcher assumed that the term "realistic job preview" would not necessarily be familiar to most supervisors. So the survey defined realistic job previews very briefly for supervisors before asking them if they used the strategy. Interestingly, fully 95% of the supervisors reported that they "tell applicants what to expect in a job, including features of the job that the person may not expect and may not like (e.g., having to work holidays or working with people who may injure them)...before the applicant decides to take the job." The most common way supervisors delivered this information was through verbal descriptions (used by 89% of the supervisors) (see Table 42). Other common preview strategies included direct observation of the people in the home (46%) and written information (35%). The average supervisor used two strategies to deliver this information. The quality and nature of the previews provided by these supervisors was not directly measured, but it appears from the strategies selected that a minority provided a thorough RJP as described by Wanous (1989). One indication of this was that only 51% of supervisors reported providing job descriptions to applicants before hiring them. Because providing a job description is an important component of an RJP, this suggests that, at best, the strategies used fell short of full explication of the technique. On the other hand, when provided with a brief description of RJPs, most supervisors recognized the strategy as something they used in some form. These findings suggest that supervisors include some information needed for a realistic job preview, but additional analysis of job preview practices would be needed to address whether comprehensive and adequately structured RJPs are being used.

Table 43. Agency Strategies to Address Staffing Problems (Time 1)

Strategies	% of Supervisors Reporting
Encourage team work among staff	80%
Manage in a way perceived by staff to be fair/ treat staff fairly	65%
Communicate clear, understandable program objectives and agency philosophy	61%
Establish effective communication among staff	45%
Use clear and understandable job roles and responsibilities	34%
Provide competitive pay and benefits	30%
Provide realistic information about the job to applicants	25%
Communicate the importance of each staff member to the agency	25%
Support the staff members	23%
Provide employee autonomy in their jobs, encourage creativity	23%
Provide staff recognition	19%
Provide a mechanism for complaints to management	16%
Use a participatory management structure	15%
Train supervisors to provide effective supervision to increase staff satisfaction with supervision	10%
Hire specific types of people/ask new hires for a time commitment	9%
Use a decentralized management structure—limit agency hierarchy	5%
Establish social involvement among employees	2%
Provide employee fitness and wellness programs	1%

$N = 110$ homes

Another strategy was used to determine the relative importance of realistic job previews as a strategy to address recruitment and retention challenges. Supervisors were asked to rank the importance of strategies they used to address staffing problems in their homes by identifying the five most important strategies they used (see Table 43). The most frequently identified strategies included encouraging team work among staff members (80% of all homes), managing fairly/treating staff members fairly (65%), communicating clear, understandable program objectives and agency philosophy (61%), establishing effective communication among staff members (45%), and establishing and communicating clear and understandable job roles and responsibilities (34%). Providing realistic job information was a priority strategy for only 25% of the supervisors.

An exploratory analysis was conducted to learn whether the strategies considered most important for addressing recruitment

Table 44. Crude Separation Rate in Homes Where the Supervisor Reported Using Particular Management Strategies

Management Practices at Time 1	Turnover @ Time 1			Turnover @ Time 2		
	No[1]	Yes	F	No[1]	Yes	F
Use direct observations to provide realistic job information to recruits	38%	51%	3.84*	48%	49%	0.02
Most effective management practice:						
Encourage team work among staff	43%	46%	0.01	45%	50%	0.21
Manage in a way that is fair	56%	40%	6.16*	57%	44%	2.10
Communicate clear, understandable program objectives and agency philosophy	45%	45%	0.01	54%	45%	1.13
Establish effective communication among staff members	42%	48%	0.74	45%	53%	0.85
Provide realistic information about the job to applicants	40%	61%	7.54**	44%	60%	2.99

$* p < .05, ** p < .01$

[1] **No** means the supervisor did not select this as one of the top five most important management strategies. **Yes** means the supervisor selected this as one of the top five strategies.

and retention challenges were associated with actual turnover rates in the homes at Time 1 and Time 2 (see Table 44). Differences in turnover rates between homes in which the supervisors did or did not rank each of the top strategies as one of the five most important strategies to them were tested using one-way analysis of variance. The use of direct observation to provide realistic information to recruits, and the selection of providing realistic information about the job to applicants as an important strategy were also tested. Of the four management practices identified by supervisors as being most effective, only one was related to turnover. Supervisors who selected managing in a fair manner/treating workers fairly as one of their five most important strategies to address staffing issues worked in homes with significantly lower turnover rates (40%) than supervisors who did not select fairness as a priority strategy (56%), F $(1, 94) = 6.16, p < .05$. Interestingly, homes that used direct observation RJPs and homes that reported providing realistic information to recruits as an important technique had significantly higher turnover rates than the other homes (51% vs. 38% for homes using direct observations vs. homes that did not, F $(1, 94) = 3.84, p < .05$; and 61% vs. 40% for supervisors reporting realistic information as an important management strategy vs. supervisors who did not, $F (1, 108) = 7.54, p$ $< .01$). It could be that supervisors in homes with higher turnover rates were more focused on the recruitment process and direct observations because recent leavers said the job was not what they expected, or it could be that an emphasis on realistic job previews is associated with less focus on strategies associated with lower turnover rates. Previous research clearly suggests that using carefully designed RJPs can reduce turnover among new hires. Therefore, this question should be explored in a study that focuses more directly on controlled testing of the effects of specific interventions on turnover rates before conclusions about its usefulness in community residential settings.

Qualitative Analysis of the Opinions of Supervisors About Recruitment and Retention Issues

Supervisors who completed the Time 2 survey were asked four open-ended questions related to the study and about their recruitment and retention practices. This section highlights the responses they provided. For this section, all Time 2 and short survey responses were included whether or not the home was qualified for the quantitative analysis described above. Therefore, the total number of surveys included in this section is 138.

Changes Influencing Recruitment, Retention, or Training

Supervisors were asked to describe any changes that had taken place in the agency or in their house that might have had an impact on the staffing outcomes addressed by this study (see Table 45). Of the supervisors who identified specific changes, the most common changes reported were a new supervisor introduced into the house (12% of all homes), staff recruitment or retention problems such as a lack of qualified applicants (10% of homes), changes in the support needs of residents (9%), and changes in hiring or recruitment practices such as changing advertising strategies, using realistic job previews, or changing the person responsible for hiring new workers (8%). Other changes mentioned by more than one supervisor were improvements in staff training; improvements in management practices; changes in wages and benefits; agency expansion; scheduling changes such as increasing the number of full-time

employees; positive attitudes of staff members; changes in the people living in the home; and changes to the agency itself such as conversion to HCBS Waiver funding, new ownership, or downsizing plans.

Most Important Factors Influencing Recruitment, Retention, and Training

Supervisors identified several factors that they felt influenced their staffing outcomes (see Table 46). By far the most common factor identified by these supervisors was wages and benefits for workers (reported by 32% of all supervisors). Other important factors included flexible or fluctuating hours (14%), problems with team work or worker participation (14%), having mature, dependable workers (13%), providing good training (13%), providing consistent, effective communication for workers (12%), providing a fun or positive work environment (11%), and using innovative recruitment practices (11%). Other factors mentioned by more than one supervisor were the skills and characteristics of residents; fair treatment of employees; support and recognition for workers; supervisor training, qualifications, and style; clear expectations; agency practices such as opportunities for advancement, location, and retention experience.

How Could the Agency Help the Supervisor Do a Better Job?

The third open-ended question asked of supervisors requested suggestions for agencies about how to make their job better (see Table 47). By far the most common response was to provide more or better training (reported by 21% of all supervisors). Other common suggestions included improve agency communication (13%), use supportive management practices (12%), and improve wages and benefits for workers and supervisors (9%). Other responses offered by more than one supervisor included help with time management, hire

Table 45. Changes Influencing Recruitment, Retention, or Training (Time 2)

Category	Sample Responses	# of Homes
No changes		18
New supervisor	Supervisor resigned or was terminated New supervisor or administrator Lack of supervisor for xx months	17
Staff recruitment or retention problems	Constant staff turnove State unemployment is low Not enough qualified applicants	14
Change in support needs of residents	Increased or decreased • physical or health challenges • behavioral needs • independence	12
Hiring or recruitment procedures	Advertising in different places or different way Changed who is responsible for hiring Started using RJP in hiring	11
Staff training	Career track was implemented Better training, more thorough and organized More training	9
Change in management practices	Quality enhancement Management or policy change Increased staff recognition Empowered staff	9
Change in wages and benefits	Increased or froze wages Changed benefit package Changed bonus policy	8
Agency expansion	Agency opened new homes	7
Change in scheduling	Developed fill-in pool Increased number of staff Increased use of full-time employees	7
Positive staff attitudes	This home has consistent long term staff.	5
Change in residents	Consumers left or died New consumers moved in	5
Change in agency status	Changes in licensing (e.g., ICF-MR to Waiver) Downsizing or pending closure New owner	5
Have not had trouble with turnover	Retention has been high	5

Transportation problems	New staff have to have car that seats four people.	1
No response		23

$N = 138$ supervisors

Table 46. Most Important Factors Influencing Recruitment, Retention, and Training (Time 2)

Category	Sample Responses	# of Home
Pay and benefits	Provide good pay and benefits Wages and benefits are inadequate Wages not competitive	44
Hours	Flexible hours offered Hours are difficult to fill Workload is problem	20
Team work or worker participation	Staff get along well/don't get along well Team work/team building is important Involve staff, listen and encourage input	20
Staff characteristics	Staff are consistent and dependable Maturity of new hires	18
Training	Good, thorough training provided Need more training/off-site training	18
Communication and feedback	Consistent, appropriate feedback Effective, open communication Make sure people understand their jobs	16
Fun or positive work environment	Enjoyable working conditions Create positive, fun, and rewarding home	15
Recruitment practices	Recruiting workers through current staff Creative advertising Realistic description of job prior to hire	15
Available workforce	No available staff/competition for staff Unemployment is high	10
Resident characteristics	Consumers are well liked Resident behavior and skills	7
Fairness	Fair treatment of employees	7
Support for staff	Adequate support from supervisor Employee recognition	6
Supervisor training, qualifications, style	Well-trained, consistent supervisors Honesty and respect	6

High or clear expectations for staff	High, clear expectations	5
Agency characteristics and practices	Opportunities for advancement Availability of transportation	5
Location	House is long way from nearest city	4
Retention experiences	Having people stay Use of seasonal or short-term workers	3
No response		15

$N = 138$ supervisors

Table 47.
How Could the Agency Help the Supervisor Do a Better Job? (Time 2)

Category	Sample Responses	# of Homes
Provide training for supervisors	Provide more/better ongoing training Provide training on specific topics	29
Improve communication	Provide updates on issues impacting home Clearly delineate job expectations Encourage open communication	18
Use fair and supportive agency management practices	Provide support during crises Delegate more/less/equally to supervisors	16
Provide staffing and recruitment support	Establish on-call pool Increase flexibility to address recruitment Don't hire before background checks are in Provide more or better applicants/staff	15
Improve wages and benefits	Improve wages and benefits for staff Improve wages and benefits for supervisors	13
Help with time management	Provide more time to do job Give time off when needed	12
Hire additional support staff	Hire more trainers, support staff, clerical assistance, human relations staff	10
Support supervisor decision making	Support supervisor decisions Trust in our judgment	9
Reduce documentation requirements	Require less paper work Provide better computer access	7
Miscellaneous	Advocate for consumers Change agency funding ICI should send results to homes	7
Address funding or budget issues	Resolve funding issues Provide better information about funding	5

Improve training for staff	Increase and improve staff training	4
Provide incentives to workers	Offer incentives for work performance	4
Improve work space	Provide office or private space Improve home maintenance	3
No response		22
No change is needed	The agency is doing a fine job	13
Don't know	Not sure	5

$N = 138$ supervisors

Table 48. Effect of Study on the Home (Time 2)

Category	Sample Responses	# of Home
None/no effect	No major effect noted	48
No response		31
Time consuming	I feel bad because I haven't been able to do it because of my time limitations. Very time consuming	18
Don't know/neutral impact	Unknown if any	14
Raised awareness/thought provoking	Doing the year's review brought to light how much of a struggle we actually did have with staffing.	13
Prompted examination and/or revision of current practices	Due to this survey I have put more thought into how people are trained and try to make it more meaningful. Makes us look at the program honestly and what we can do to improve the overall operation of our program.	7
Staff participation or follow-through lacking	Staff not always willing to participate Also, the staff doesn't follow through	5
Negative impact on home	Produces more paperwork that could have been directed at direct care. It has been somewhat of a stressor because we haven't been able to hire and you keep calling so often.	5

$N = 138$ supervisors

dditional support staff, support supervisor ecision making, reduce documentation equirements, address funding and budget- ng issues, improve training for direct upport workers, provide incentives for orkers, and improve work space for upervisors.

What Effect Did This Study Have on the Home?

The final open-ended question asked upervisors to report any positive or negative ffects of the study on the home (see Table 48). Most supervisors (67%) reported the study had no impact, did not answer the question, or reported that the impact was neutral. Of those who did report an impact the most common impact was that the study took much time (13% of supervisors). Other supervisors reported that the study raised their awareness of turnover issues (9%) and that the study prompted examination or revision of current practices (5%). Five supervisors reported negative impacts of the study on the home generally related to the time demands of the study.

CHAPTER 6

STUDY 2 RESULTS:
THE STUDY OF NEWLY HIRED
DIRECT SUPPORT WORKERS

Individual direct support workers provided information about their characteristics and experiences at several points during the study. Analyses focused on those characteristics and experiences reported at hire and after 30 days by direct support workers who stayed in the home, were promoted or moved to another house in the same agency (stayers), and direct support workers who voluntarily resigned their positions (leavers). Workers who were fired were excluded except in the open-ended responses.

Personal Characteristics of Direct Support Participants

There were no differences between stayers and leavers in personal and job characteristics (see Table 49). Newly hired workers were predominantly female (81%) and were 28.8 years old at hire. Newly hired workers were overwhelmingly white (96%), unmarried (75%), with no financial dependents (76%). New hires had an average of 1.9 years of experience in developmental disabilities and had completed one and a half years of post-

Table 49. Personal and Job Characteristics of Stayers and Leavers

Characteristic	Stayers	Leavers	Mean *(SD)/* % of DSWs
Female	79%	83%	81%
Age at hire	28.6	29.1	28.8 (10.5)
Ethnic Background			
White	97%	96%	96%
Black	0%	2%	1%
Hispanic	0%	2%	1%
American Indian, Alaskan Native	3%	0%	2%
Married	24%	26%	25%
With financial dependents	26%	21%	24%
Years of experience in the field	2.0	1.8	1.9 (3.1)
Years of school	13.5	13.8	13.6 (2.0)
Have taken courses on mental retardation	42%	31%	37%
Currently in voc./tech. school or college	19%	21%	20%

N = 105 direct support workers (58 stayers, 47 leavers)
None of the differences between stayers and leavers were statistically significant.

Table 50. Recruitment Experiences: Source of Job Information

Characteristic	Stayers	Leavers	Mean (SD)/ % DSWs	F/X²
Media advertisement (TV, radio, newspaper)	31%	51%	40%	17.4*
Current/former employee of this agency	43%	21%	33%	
A friend who works at a similar agency	12%	6%	10%	
Other	7%	2%	5%	
Explored possibility on my own initiative	3%	2%	3%	
High school or college placement office	3%	2%	3%	
Employment or referral agency	0%	6%	3%	
Person with DD or family member	0%	4%	2%	
Worked for agency before	0%	4%	2%	
Used "inside sources"	57%	36%	47% (.50)	4.34*
Saw job description before hire	71%	69%	70% (.46)	0.02

* $p < .05$, $N = 105$ direct support workers (58 stayers, 47 leavers)

secondary education at hire. Approximately one third (37%) of all new hires had taken a course on mental retardation, and 20% were currently enrolled in a postsecondary educational program. Among the participants who had not worked for the present agency before starting in this home, stayers had 2.0 prior years of experience while leavers had 1.8 years of experience. None of these differences were statistically significant.

Recruitment Experiences

There were significant differences between stayers and leavers in the most important source of information about the job (see Table 50). Specifically, leavers were more likely to use outside sources (such as media advertisements or employment or referral agencies), while stayers were more likely to use inside sources (such as a current or former employee of this agency or a friend who works at a similar agency) to find out about the job, $F(1, 94) = 4.34$, $p < .05$. This finding is consistent with other research on recruitment sources.

There were no significant differences between stayers and leavers regarding why they took the job (see Table 51). Overall 36% said they took the job primarily because they needed the income or benefits provided; 35% of new hires said they took the job because they had a special interest in the home or people in the home; and 17% took the job because they needed the training or experience for their careers.

Job Characteristics

There were no significant differences between stayers and leavers in the general characteristics of their jobs (see Table 52). The average new hire worked 26.1 hours per week, which included four weekend shifts in an average month. Most new hires worked the 3:00 P.M. to 11:00 P.M. shift (61%). A few worked mornings (17%) or awake (19%) or asleep (3%) overnight shifts. Overall 7% of

Table 51. Most Important Reason for Taking the Job

Characteristic	Stayers	Leavers	% of DSWs	X^2
I needed the income or benefits provided.	35%	38%	36%	2.34
I have a special interest in the home or people in the home.	31%	40%	35%	
The job provided needed training or experience.	21%	13%	17%	
Other	14%	9%	11%	

N = 105 direct support workers (58 stayers, 47 leavers)

Table 52. Job Characteristics of Stayers and Leavers

Characteristic	Stayers	Leavers	Mean (SD)/ % or DSWs	SD
Hours worked per week	28.1	23.7	26.1	12.7
Weekend days worked per month	4.2	4.0	4.1	2.0
Primary shift				
7:00 A.M. to 3:00 P.M.	21%	13%	17%	
3:00 P.M. to 11:00 P.M.	59%	64%	61%	
11:00 P.M. to 7:00 A.M. - awake	17%	21%	19%	
11:00 P.M. to 7:00 A.M. - asleep	3%	2%	3%	
Live at the home	5%	9%	7%	0.3
Current hourly wage	$7.22	$6.82	$7.04	$1.52
Overall contrast of pay at this job with wants/needs[1]	7.7	7.5	7.6	1.8
Years plan to stay	3.9	3.2	3.6	5.3

N = 105 direct support workers (58 stayers, 47 leavers)

None of the differences between stayers and leavers were statistically significant.

[1]The scale measured the discrepancy between pay vs. what I want, pay vs. previous job, and pay vs. need (1 = the job provides much more, 5 = the job provides much less)

newly hired workers lived at the home in which they worked. The average starting salary for new workers was $7.04 per hour. Stayers and leavers reported an average score of 7.6 of 15 points possible on the extent to which their pay matched what they wanted and needed. A higher score suggests that the job does not match the salary needs of the new hire. The average new hire planned to work in the home for 3.6 years.

Job Expectations

Stayers and leavers did not differ in how much they reported knowing about the job at hire (see Table 53). Likewise stayers or leavers did not differ in the proportion who saw a job description before they were hired. Overall new hires reported knowing most about the types of tasks they would be doing, their pay and benefits, and the needs and characteristics of the people living in the homes. They knew least about the agency's reputation and about what other direct support workers would be like.

New direct support workers rated 21 job characteristics from the Minnesota Satisfaction Questionnaire (see Table 54) and 6 items regarding support and assistance in terms of (a) the extent to which they expected the feature to be present in their new job (see Table 55) and (b) how important each characteristic is to them. The rankings of expectations and importance were very similar. Among the items on the MSQ, newly hired workers reported the most important features were: having a chance to do things for other people, having a good boss, having

a supervisor who is competent in making decisions, having a job that would provide steady employment, having work that would not go against their conscience, and having a job that provided a feeling of accomplishment. Usually, workers were satisfied to very satisfied with these features after 30 days on the job.

As for expectations about support and assistance available, the most important features were that the supervisor would provide advice and support, that backup support would be available for emergencies, and that training and technical assistance would be available (see Table 55). As with the MSQ items, workers were generally satisfied after 30 days with these job features.

Job Experiences and Outcome

Employment Context

Once study participants had been in their jobs for at least 30 days, they were surveyed to find out about their initial job experience and attitudes (see Table 56). Overall new hires reported engaging in 1.5 of 10 listed jo

Table 53. Prehire Knowledge of Stayers and Leavers

Knowledge and Expectation	Stayers	Leavers	Mean	SD
Types of tasks you would be doing	3.6	3.4	3.5	1.2
Your pay and benefits	3.0	3.1	3.1	1.2
Characteristics of people in the home	2.9	3.1	3.0	1.4
Working conditions in this home	2.8	2.8	2.8	1.3
What your supervisor would be like	2.8	2.7	2.8	1.5
Agency reputation	2.7	2.2	2.5	1.3
What the other workers would be like	2.6	2.3	2.3	1.3
Overall average	2.9	2.7	2.8	1.0

1 = nothing, 5 = a great deal
N = 105 direct support workers (58 stayers, 47 leavers)
The overall average scores for stayers and leavers did not vary significantly.

Table 54. Job Expectations of Newly Hired Direct Support Workers (Based on the MN Satisfaction Questionnaire)

Expectation at Hire	Expect Feature[a] N = 174	Feature Is Important[a] N = 174	Satisfaction at 30 Days[b] N = 138
I will have a chance to do things for other people.	1.4	1.5	4.6
I will have a good boss.	1.6	1.4	4.0
My supervisor will be competent in making decisions.	1.6	1.4	4.1
My job will provide steady employment.	1.7	1.5	4.3
I will be doing things that do not go against my conscience.	1.8	1.5	4.3
I will get a feeling of accomplishment from the job.	1.8	1.5	4.0
I will be able to do different things from time to time.	1.8	1.7	4.1
I will be doing things that use my abilities.	1.8	1.7	4.0
My co-workers will get along together.	1.9	1.5	4.0
I will be satisfied with the working conditions.	1.9	1.6	4.2
I will have freedom to use my own judgment.	1.9	1.8	4.0
I will be able to work independently.	2.0	2.0	4.2
I will like the way company policies are put into practice.	2.1	1.9	3.7
I will get praise for doing a good job.	2.2	1.9	3.8
I will be able to keep busy all the time.	2.2	2.0	4.0
I will be respected by the community.	2.2	2.2	3.5
I will be satisfied with my pay and the amount of work I do.	2.3	1.9	3.5
I will have chances for advancement on this job.	2.4	2.0	3.4
I will be able to try my own methods of doing the job.	2.5	2.2	3.8
I will have a chance to tell other people what to do.	3.1	3.4	3.1

[a] 1 = strongly agree, 5 = strongly disagree
[b] 1 = very dissatisfied, 5 = very satisfied

Table 55. Expectations of New Direct Support Workers Regarding Support and Assistance Available

Expectation at Hire	Expect Feature[a] N = 174	Feature Is Important[a] N = 174	Satisfaction at 30 Days[b] N = 138
My supervisor will provide advice and support.	1.6	1.5	4.2
Backup support will be available for emergencies.	1.7	1.4	4.1
Training and technical assistance will be available.	1.7	1.5	4.0
Adequate equipment and supplies will be available.	1.7	1.6	3.9
Adequate money and transportation will be available for community activities.	1.7	1.7	4.0
My fellow workers will provide advice and support.	1.8	1.6	4.1

[a]1 = strongly agree, 5 = strongly disagree
[b]1 = very dissatisfied, 5 = very satisfied

Table 56. Employment Context After 30 Days

Factor	Stayers (N)	Leavers (N)	Total (SD)	F
Number of job search activities	1.2 (58)	1.9 (47)	1.5 (2.0)	2.14
Quality of other job opportunities[b]	12.1 (48)	13.3 (36)	12.6 (3.4)	2.61
Likelihood of being promoted[a]	3.0 (48)	1.3 (36)	1.8 (1.3)	9.98**
Likelihood of being laid off[a]	1.7 (48)	1.7 (36)	1.7 (1.2)	0.01

**$p < .01$
[a]1 = highly unlikely, 7 = highly likely
[b]1 = excellent, 5 = terrible

search activities. There were no statistically significant differences between stayers and leavers in the quality of other jobs available to them. The workers scored an average of 12.6 points on a scale that ranged to 20, with 20 suggesting that alternative job opportunities are excellent compared with this job. Stayers and leavers differed significantly in the likelihood of being promoted. Stayers thought their chances of being promoted were significantly better (3.0 on a scale of 5) compared with leavers (who scored 1.3 on the same scale), $F(1, 82) = 9.98, p < .01$.

Stayers and leavers reported that it was very unlikely that they would be laid off from their current positions (scoring an average of 1.7 points on a scale ranging from 1= highly unlikely to 7 = highly likely).

Job Outcomes

After 30 days, stayers and leavers differed on several job outcomes (see Table 57). They differed on how likely it was that they would leave their position, the extent of their commitment to the organization, and the extent to which the job met their original

Table 57. Job Outcomes for New Direct Support Workers After 30 Days

Outcome	Stayers (N = 48)	Leavers (N = 36)	Total (SD)	F/X^2
Current salary	$7.38	$6.93	$7.19 ($1.60)	1.63
Intent to leave	19.2	25.5	21.9 (11.2)	6.92**
Organizational commitment	83.0	74.9	79.5 (11.6)	11.07***
Job responsibilities/work conditions turned out to be what I expected[a]	1.7	1.9	1.8 (1.1)	0.64
Overall does this job meet original expectations[a]	1.6	2.2	1.8 (1.0)	7.03**
Job Satisfaction (MSQ)	80.2	77.0	78.8 (9.3)	2.49
Intrinsic Satisfaction (MSQ)	48.5	47.3	48.0 (5.4)	1.04
Extrinsic Satisfaction (MSQ)	23.5	21.4	22.6 (4.0)	5.88*
Satisfaction with supports and resources	24.5	24.3	24.4 (3.8)	0.48

$*p < .05, **p < .01, ***p < .001$
[a] 1 = definitely yes, 5 = definitely no

overall expectations. Leavers were more likely to say they planned or intended to leave, $F(1, 82) = 6.92, p < .01$, reported less organizational commitment, $F(1, 82) = 11.07, p < .001$), and were less likely to say the job met their original expectations overall, $F(1, 81) = 7.03, p < .01$. There were no differences between stayers and leavers in salary after 30 days, in the extent to which the actual job responsibilities were as expected, or in whether they received adequate co-worker support. As for job satisfaction, there were no overall differences in job satisfaction, but leavers did report significantly less satisfaction with externally related job factors (e.g., pay for the amount of work, praise for doing a good job) than stayers did, $F(1, 82) = 5.88, p < .05$). The groups did not differ in their satisfaction with supports and resources available to them.

Training, Socialization, and Supervision Experiences

Several sets of questions were used to determine satisfaction of new hires with training, socialization, and supervision practices during their first 30 days on the job. Stayers and leavers reported similar types experiences in all of these areas (see Table 58).

Overall new workers agreed that the orientation and training they recieved had met their needs (31.2 of 40 points on 8 questions). Organizational socialization practices were measured using five questions in each of six areas. Both stayers and leavers reported socialization experiences that were mostly group or collective (new workers go through a similar set of group experiences); formal (new workers are separated from the regular workforce during initial socialization); sequential (the order in which training will occur is clear to the new worker); fixed (timelines for completing various stages such as probation are clear); serial (experienced workers act as role models for new recruits); and investiture focused (current workers provide positive social support to new workers) (descriptions from Jones, 1986). Both stayers and leavers reported that they recieved substantial support from

Table 58. Training and Supervision Experience for New Direct Support Workers in First 30 Days

Factor	Stayers (*N*)	Leavers(*N*)	Mean	SD
Training experiences	31.6 (44)	30.7 (37)	31.2	4.5
Organizational socialization practices [a] *N*=43		*N*=30		
Group vs. individual training	23.6	23.0	23.4	6.2
Formal vs. informal training	21.1	22.8	21.8	4.7
Sequential vs. random training	22.5	21.2	22.0	4.6
Fixed vs. variable training	20.3	19.4	19.9	4.4
Disjunctive vs. serial training	17.4	18.5	17.8	4.1
Investiture training	21.7	21.2	21.5	4.0
Co-worker support for socialization	33.4	31.3	32.5	5.4
Leader Behavior Description Questionnaire				
Initiating structure	40.0 (41)	42.6 (35)	41.1	7.7
Consideration	43.9 (41)	43.7 (32)	43.8	9.4
Overall supervisor rating	13.0 (43)	13.3 (37)		
Support from interdisciplinary team				
Treated as important and equal member of[b] ID team	2.1(44)	2.1(37)	2.1	1.2
Supported by case managers and staff from[b] other programs	1.8(44)	1.9(37)	1.8	1.0

[a] A score of 20 on organizational practices indicates training that is balanced between the polar extremes listed. Score above 20 indicates training more like the first characteristic listed, while a score below 20 indicates training more like the second characteristic.
[b] 1 = definitely yes, 5 = definitely no
None of the differences between stayers and leavers were statistically significant.

current workers during socialization (reporting 32.5 of 42 possible points on the scale) with the differences between stayers and leavers not reaching statistical significance.

Scores on the Leader Behavior Description Questionnaire were divided into two components. Supervisors in this study had Initiating Structure scores of 41.1 of 60 possible points with higher scores indicating a supervisor provides more structure to the work group. Initiating Structure is measured using 15 items such as making attitudes clear to the group, criticizing poor work, emphasizing meeting deadlines, and asks that group members follow standard rules and regulations. For comparison, military aircraft commanders with an average of eight crew members scored 41.6 on this item while educational administrators supervising an average of seven staff members scored 37.9 points (Halpin, 1957). Differences between stayers and leavers were not statistically significant.

The other component of the Leader Behavior Description Questionnaire was the rating by new hires of their supervisors on consideration. New hires reported their supervisors scored an average of 43.8 points of 60 possible in this scale with higher scores indicating a supervisor who is more consider-ate of the individual needs and characteristics of workers. The consideration scale included 15 items such as doing personal favors for group members, finding time to listen to group members, and treating all group members as equals. For comparison, military aircraft commanders scored an average of 41.4 points and educational administrators scored an average of 44.7 points on this scale (Halpin, 1957).

The supervisor rating measured how often (1 meaning never and 5 meaning always) the supervisor made good decisions about the work schedule, made good decisions about resident training and programs, and looked out for the welfare of residents. Both stayers and leavers said their supervisors often to always engaged in these basic behaviors.

Table 59. Survival Rates of New Hires in Small Group Homes

# of Months	# Stayed in Position	% in Same Position	# Promoted	# Lateral Move	# Left Voluntarily	# Terminated
At hire	124	100%				
0	119	96%	0	1	3	1
1	109	88%	0	1	5	4
2	100	81%	0	2	5	2
3	87	70%	1	3	5	4
4	81	65%	1	1	3	1
5	75	61%	0	3	3	0
6	70	57%	0	0	2	3
7	64	52%	0	0	4	2
8	61	49%	0	0	3	0
9	57	46%	0	0	4	0
10	52	42%	0	1	3	1
11	48	39%	0	0	4	0
12	41	33%	2	1	3	1
Total	41	33%	4 (3%)	13 (11%)	47 (38%)	19 (15%)

Finally, new workers reported that they felt they were treated as an important and equal member of the interdisciplinary team, and that they received the support they needed from case managers and staff from other programs to be as effective as they would like with the residents. Again, there were no differences between stayers and leavers.

Survival Rates

Survival rates are reported for the 124 people whose status at 12 months was known, and who were new to the agency and the home at the time they were hired (see Table 59). In all, 33% of newly hired workers remained in their positions for at least 12 months. An additional 3% were promoted within the agency, and 11% made a lateral move to another service site. On the other hand, 38% of all new hires voluntarily resigned their positions within 12 months, while 15% of all new hires were terminated during that period. From the perspective of the people with developmental disabilities living in these homes, more than half the new workers who entered their lives to support them were no longer doing so 8 months later.

The timing of leaving varied depending on the type of leaving. Of the new hires who made a lateral move, most (85%) made the move within the first 5 months on the job. Just over half the new hires who left volun-

Table 60. Supervisor Exit Questionnaire: Differences Between Various Types of Leavers

| Question | TYPE OF EXIT | | | | Total | F |
| | Promoted | Lateral Move | Left Voluntarily | Terminated | | |
	$N = 5$	$N = 20$	$N = 57$	$N = 20$	$N = 102$	
Would you rehire this person?[a]	4.6	4.4	3.8	1.6	3.5	18.5***
Job performance of leaver?[b]	4.4	4.0	3.7	2.0	3.5	17.5***
Voluntariness of leaving?[c]	20.2	22.0	22.9	22.8	22.6	2.3
Avoidability of leaving?[d]	21.6	19.9	20.4	23.1	20.9	5.0**
How hard to replace this person with someone who will do as good a job?[e]	3.6	3.4	3.3	2.3	3.1	7.3***
Will person continue on-call hours?	20%	40%	16%	0%	18%	4.1***

** $p < .01$, *** $p < .001$
This table includes all leavers whether they were new to the agency or not.
[a] 1 = under no circumstances, 5 = definitely
[b] 1 = inadequate, 5 = excellent
[c] Higher scores indicate that the person had more choice in whether they left.
[d] Higher scores indicate that the supervisor had more control over whether a person left.
[e] 1 = very easy, 5 = very difficult

tarily did so in the first 6 months. Of the new hires who were terminated, 79% were fired in the first 6 months on the job.

Supervisor Exit Questionnaire Results

Supervisors completed exit surveys for all direct support participants who left the home during the study. All leavers, whether or not they were new to the agency at the time they began working in a study home, are included on Table 60. These variables were analyzed using a one-way analysis of variance with Student-Neuman-Kuhls follow-up tests. There were significant differences between workers who left voluntarily (for another position in the agency or for a job outside the agency) and those who were fired from their positions involuntarily. Specifically, supervisors were significantly less willing to rehire those who were terminated, reported the job perfor- mance of those who were terminated was significantly lower than the others, and reported it would be much easier to replace those who had been terminated compared with those who left for other reasons. Workers who made a lateral move were more likely to remain on-call than workers who were terminated. Finally, supervisors reported that there was more supervisor control over leaving by persons who were terminated than over leaving by persons who moved laterally to another position.

Workers were counted as having left the home when they no longer had regularly scheduled hours there. A few of those who left continued to work occasional on-call hours in the studied home. This proportion ranged from 0% among those who were terminated to 40% among the direct support workers who transferred to another home.

Discriminant Analysis of Staying or Leaving

The final analysis for individual-level turnover was a discriminant analysis to identify the proportion of variability in staying or leaving

accounted for by a preselected set of variables. Based on previous research, 11 variables were selected for being related to individual-level turnover. Those variables consisted of: organizational commitment, met expectations, quality of alternative job options, current salary, job satisfaction, supervisor structure, the source of information about the job, hours worked per week, months in the field of developmental disabilities at the time of hire, age at hire, and intent to stay or leave at the time of hire. This analysis was completed on the 77 workers who were new to the agency at the time of hire, who were not fired from their positions, who had completed information about all 11 variables. Several leavers were excluded from the analysis because they left the home before completing the 30-day survey. Overall these 11 variables accounted for 26% of the variability in whether a new hire would stay for 12 months (Wilk's Lambda = .737, X^2 = 21.189, $p < .05$) (see Tables 62 and 63). Unique contributions to predicting staying or leaving were made by organizational commit- ment, level of met expectations, and perceived job opportunities (see Table 61). The classifica- tion results from this analysis correctly predicted group membership for 74% overall including correctly predicting the status of 73% of stayers and 75% of leavers (see Table 64).

Qualitative Analysis of Experiences of Newly Hired Direct Support Workers

For Leavers

Besides the quantitative data collected from new hires, workers who left their positions answered several qualitative questions at the time of the exit interview. This group included those who were promoted, those who were transferred, those who resigned, and those who were terminated. However, only 33 of 117 leavers (28%) completed the exit interview, so their responses cannot be considered to represent the sample.

Table 61. Discriminant Analysis of Factors Associated With Staying or Leaving w/in 12 Months

Independent Variables	Standardized Canonical Discriminant Function Coefficients	Pooled w/in Groups, Correlations Between Discriminating Variables & Standardized Canonical Discriminant Function	Wilk's Lambda (df 1, 75)	F
Organizational commitment	.289	.581	.893	9.01**
Overall met expectations	-.187	-.436	.937	5.08*
Alternative jobs available	-.462	-.425	.940	4.83*
Current salary	.131	.318	.965	2.71
Job Satisfaction	.414	.304	.968	2.47
Supervisor structure	-.668	-.274	.974	2.01
Inside source	.307	.265	.976	1.88
Hours worked per week	.411	.234	.981	1.47
Months in field at hire	.124	.229	.982	1.40
Age at hire	.154	-.019	1.00	0.01
Intent to leave	.552	.001	1.00	0.00

$*p < .05$, $**p < .01$, $N = 77$ newly hired direct support workers

Table 62. Summary of Canonical Discriminant Function for Staying or Leaving

Function	Eigenvalue	% of Variance	Cumulative %	Canonical Correlation
1	.356	100.0%	100.0%	.513

Table 63. Wilk's Lambda for Discriminant Function

Test of Function	Wilk's Lambda	Chi-Square	df	Sig.
1	.737	21.189	11	.031

Table 64. Classification Results for Stayers vs. Leavers

	Classification		Predicted Group Membership		
			Stayer	Leaver	Total
Original Group Membership	Count	Stayer	33	12	45
		Leaver	8	24	32
	Percent	Stayer	73%	27%	
		Leaver	25%	75%	

74% of new hours correctly classified as stayers or leavers by this equation

Table 65. Primary Reason for Decision to Leave (Leavers)

Category	Sample Responses	# of Leavers
New job with better pay or benefits.	I left for a higher paying job with benefits.	8
Promotion or transfer within company	Was offered supervisory position at another house.	5
Needed more time off	I was working too much— had another job. I had no free time when I worked weekends.	5
Wages or benefits are bad	No family health insurance Not enough pay	4
Problems with residents	Lifting of consumers Severe behavior problems	4
Personal reasons	Working with mentally handicapped persons was not what I expected. Physical health is not good	4
New job in other field	Obtained position in field of specialty	3
New job closer to home	Took a position in a new group home that was much closer to my home.	3
Problems with supervisor	The supervisor was not performing his job properly.	2
Other	School Left for Europe	2

$N = 33$ direct support worker leavers

Table 66. Type of Position You Plan to Take Next (Leavers)

Category	Sample Responses	# of Leavers
Promotion or similar position in another group home or day program	Supervisor in a group homePCA at another group home with better pay	15
Job outside human services	Factory work Senior buyer	7
Other human services position	Adolescent care worker and interpreter for the deaf LPN in a nursing home Home health aide	7
Complete education	Medical student Complete BSW	3
Unsure	No present plans	3

$N = 33$ direct support worker leavers

What Were the Primary Reasons for Leaving?

A total of 40 responses were received regarding why a person left the job from the 33 leavers who answered the survey. Of those who completed exit questionnaires, eight (24%) reported they left for a new job with better pay or benefits, five (15%) left for a promotion or transfer within the company, five (15%) left because they needed more time off. Several other reasons were mentioned by four or fewer leavers (see Table 65).

What Type of Position Will You Take Next?

Thirty-five responses were received from the 33 workers regarding their next position. Of the leavers, 15 (42% of all leavers) reported that they were moving to a promotion or a similar position, 7 (21%) said they were getting a job outside human services entirely, and 7 (21%) were taking a human service position working with another population (see Table 66).

What Would You Tell a Friend Applying for Your Job?

Leavers were also asked what they would tell their best friend about the job. Both positive and negative job characteristics were mentioned (see Table 67). The most common positive features mentioned included the residents are great (reported by 30% of leavers), the co-workers are great (18%), and it is a rewarding job (15%). The most common negative characteristics mentioned included the job duties can be difficult or demanding (36% of leavers), the pay, benefits or chances for advancement are not great (18%), the supervisor in this house is bad (15%), and the hours are bad (15%).

Describe an Incident That Made You Decide to Leave.

Leavers were also asked to describe the incident(s) that made them decide to leave the job. Responses are provided in general categories in Table 68. The most frequently mentioned incidents were related to an offer or decision to get a better job (30%). Other critical incidents related to the need for more money or better benefits (18%), and better relationships with supervisor (18%). About one quarter of leavers could think of no specific incident (24%).

Table 67. Advice to Potential Employees (Leavers)

Category	Sample Responses	# of Leavers
Negative characteristics		
Job duties can be difficult or demanding	Sometimes the care can be gross. The night shift is physically hard (lifting). Stressful situations (medical, behavior)	12
The pay/benefits and chances for advancement are not great	There are better jobs for the same or better pay. The potential for improving or moving up isn't there.	6
The supervisor is bad	Take another house, supervisor. The house supervisor is difficult to get along with.	5
The hours are bad	The hours fluctuate 16 to 40 hours per week.	5
Co-workers are difficult	Keep to yourself because of secrets.	3
Other	It's a long drive. Company is not experienced in handling severe behavior problems.	3
Positive characteristics		
The residents are great	You'll enjoy working with the consumers and their great personalities.	10
The co-workers are great	Very friendly, respectable home Staff are wonderful to work with	6
It's a rewarding job	This job makes you feel like you're really doing something worthwhile.	5
Need to be a patient person	You must have a great deal of patience.	4
The pay/benefits or chance for advancement are good	Above average pay There are opportunities for advancement.	4
The company is good	I like the organization Good people to work for	4
The supervisor is good	QMRP is great to work with. Supervisor is very considerate.	3
The hours are good	Easy hours	2
Other	Stress communication upon taking the position. You really have to want to be in this position.	4

N = 33 direct support worker leavers

Table 68. Incidents That Made You Want to Leave (Leavers)

Category	Sample Responses	# of Leavers
Got or decided to get a better job	Long drive, I had an opportunity to better myself with another job. A job in my field of training	10
Need more money or better benefits	Purely left due to health benefits An opportunity to make more money	6
Supervisor issues	Ineffective communication between staff and house supervisor	6
Problems with duties	Strenuous physical labor I had to floss teeth	3
Challenging behavior	One of the residents yelled at me and slammed a door in my face.	3
Schedule was difficult	Feeling exhausted; not enough time for myself.	2
Issues with co-worker	People were talking about me behind my back.	1
Nothing/no response	It had nothing to do with any incidents.	8

N = 33 direct support worker leavers

What Could the Agency Have Done to Make You Stay?

The final question for leavers asked what the agency could have done to make the person stay (see Table 69). Most leavers (61%) reported that there was nothing the agency could have done, because the job was not a good match or it was time to move on. Other responses included offer more money or better benefits (27%), change the staffing patterns or process (12%), or support or supervise the workers better (12%).

All Workers at 30 Days, 6 Months, and 12 Months

A second set of questions was asked of workers who remained in their positions. The questions were asked at 30 days, at 6 months, and again at 12 months of employment. Responses from all three surveys combined were used to develop the categories. If a staff member reported the same answer on two or more surveys, that person was counted only once for this analysis. The maximum number of responses in this set of questions is 138, the number of workers who completed a survey at 30 days after hire.

Describe an Incident That Made You Decide to Stay

A first step in creating a realistic job preview is to identify, from the perspective of current employees, the most salient characteristics of the job, both positive and negative. Several questions asked of stayers addressed these issues. The first question for stayers was what incidents made them decide they wanted to stay on the job (see Table 70). The most common response, provided by 57 workers (41%), was "I enjoy the people who live in this house." Examples in this category included, "The clients are the best," "They get me to laugh," and "I enjoy working with the clients." Other common responses included that they liked the co-workers (35%), and that they felt the people who live in the home needed or appreciated the worker (35%). Other workers liked the pay or benefits (24%), the supervisor (21%), or the hours (18%).

Table 69. What Could Agency Have Done to Make You Stay? (Leavers)

Category	Sample Responses	# of Leavers
Nothing	Realistically, almost nothing Nothing! It is not my field of expertise. It's time for me to move on.	20
More money or benefits	Offered more money Give me grants for school to move up in the job	9
Change staffing patterns	Use a better hiring/firing process Create a FT position in this cottage	4
Support or supervise staff better	More transfer training More support from upper management Hire a new house supervisor Change dramatically the way they ran the company.	4

$N = 33$ direct support worker leavers

Describe an Incident That Made You Want to Leave.

Workers were also asked to identify incidents that made them want to leave the home or quit the job (see Table 71). More than half of the workers (51%) said there were no incidents that made them want to leave, and another 23% did not respond to the question. Of those who did identify issues, the most common incidents were problems with co-workers such as staff talking behind each other's back (17%), inadequate pay, benefits, or incentives (16%), problems with supervisors (13%), and scheduling problems (13%).

What Could Your Employer Do to Make Your Job Better?

Another way to begin analyzing what strategies might be useful to address staffing issues is to ask the workers what the employer could do to make the job better. Overwhelmingly, the most common response was to increase or improve pay, benefits, or other incentives (37%) (see Table 72). Another 33% of workers said no changes were needed because the employer or supervisor was doing a good job already. Other common suggestions included asking the supervisor to be more personable and attentive and to do a better, job managing the home (17%), or to give the workers more, better, or different hours (17%).

What Was the Hardest Thing When You Started This Job?

Although socialization practices experienced by direct support workers did not predict differences between stayers and leavers, new workers identified several ways to make the organizational entry process easier or more effective. When new workers were asked to report what the hardest part of starting their job was, two responses were most common (see Table 73). Workers reported they had difficulty getting to know the people living in the home and their behaviors and traits. This response was reported by 45% of all new hires. The other common response, reported by 43% of new hires, was that learning the routines and duties was difficult. A smaller but still substantial group of new workers reported having difficulty getting to know and get along with other staff members (20%) and adjusting to the work schedule, particularly for those who worked overnight or early morning shifts (14%).

Table 70. Incidents That Made You Decide to Stay

Category	Sample Responses	# of DSWs
I enjoy the people who live in this house.	Consumers are the best. They get me to laugh. Enjoy working with the consumers	57
I like my co-workers	I enjoy my fellow workers. Having competent co-workers	49
The people who live here like me/ need me/appreciate me.	Being able to help them and understand them Having a consumer ask me to sit with her	48
Money or benefits	Great pay and benefits Overtime is offered almost every pay period.	33
I like my supervisor.	I have a wonderful supervisor. The supervisor supports staff decisions.	29
The hours work well for me.	I can work two jobs. The hours are great.	25
The staff are team players.	Everyone works together well. Supportive interactions with co-workers	17
I like the atmosphere or working environment.	Good working conditions I like working in a small home.	16
I like the company.	The agency cares about the residents. Good programs are implemented.	16
I enjoy this job or line of work.	I enjoy the job I perform. I feel satisfied with my job.	15
Activities with the residents	Being able to take the consumers out to eat Taking the residents to see fireworks on July 4th	12
Offers steady convenient employment	Enjoy job security It's close to my home.	12
Offers opportunities for input, challenge, and independence	I like to work alone. I'm often asked for input.	11
The people are easy to care for.	Consumers get along well New house with only 4 people.	9
I am adjusting to the job.	Program members are getting to know me. Getting used to the routine and consumers	4
I don't like the job or parts of it.	Can't get another job with promotion Filing a vulnerable adult report	4
None	Can't think of any right now	9
No response		11

$N = 138$ newly hired direct support workers

Table 71. Incidents That Made You Want to Leave

Category	Sample Responses	# of DSWs
Problems with co-workers	Staff talk behind each other's backs. Shifts pitting against each other gets stressful. Performance of certain employees	24
Inadequate pay/benefits or incentives	Not enough money Total lack of incentive Lack of benefits	22
Problems with supervisor	The supervisor is unfair. Supervisor didn't follow through. Lack of communication and support from supervisor	18
Scheduling problems	Tired of working overnights, tired of weekends Need more hours	18
Behavior of residents	Residents screaming and drooling Verbal and physical abuse from aggressive residents Self-injurious behaviors	13
Dislike duties	Toileting accidents Too much work Physical duties too difficult	12
Objection to company programs or treatment of consumers	Treatment of residents by certain staff I have a lot of energy and just sit around Lack of good planning for healthy menus	11
Better job	Change of career Promotion	8
Lack of mobility in company	Little or no chance of promotion	5
Other	Had to take a lot of intense training Got a vulnerable adult report against me but I wasn't in the building when it happened. Lack of privacy as live-in My 20 some years are in Location Always being short of staff	13
None/I don't plan to leave	Nothing. I like my job.	70
No response		32

N = 138 newly hired direct support workers

Table 72. What Could Your Employer Do to Make Your Job Better?

Category	Sample Responses	# of DSW
Increase or improve pay, benefits, or other incentives	Pay me more money Give merit raises Better benefits Bonuses for jobs well done	51
No changes are needed	Nothing. He is doing a great job.	46
Be more personable and attentive/ Do a better job managing the home	Be more involved — deal with staff issues Follow through on his plans Be more attentive to staff Be available to staff more often	24
Give me more, better, or different hours	More weekends off Give me more hours Be more consistent with the schedule	24
Improve communication with staff/Provide more feedback	Let me know that I am valued as an employee Communicate better Do more frequent evaluations	19
Provide more or better training	More hands-on training in the beginning Provide 1:1 training	18
Provide enough staff	Fully staff homes before opening new ones Employ more people	9
Treat staff equally, address discipline issues	Be more fair to all staff Be more strict on people who don't do their job Fire or suspend employees	8
Create more opportunities to move up	Have more chance for advancement Give me more responsibility	6
Provide resources needed	Provide money for supplies, groceries, equipment	4
Make home improvements	Upgrade accessibility of home	3
Schedule more activities for home	Have more to do in the evenings	3
Reduce paperwork	Get rid of repetitive paperwork	2
Change who lives in the home	Add another person to the home	2
No response		24

$N = 138$ newly hired direct support workers

Table 73. What Was the Hardest Part as You Started This Job?

Category	Sample Responses	# of DSWs
Getting to know the people in the home and their behaviors and traits	Getting to know everyone Getting to know their different personalities Learning and dealing with behaviors Learning consumer's needs and abilities	62
Learning the routines and completing my duties	Getting used to the routine Learning specific procedures and programs Learning my way around the kitchen	59
Getting to know the other staff members/Finding that not everyone gets along with one another	Getting to know the staff Dealing with staff not getting along Trying to adjust to new staff all the time	28
Adjusting to the schedule	Getting used to the hours Staying awake at night	20
Learning and remembering everything	Learning everything so fast Remembering the small details	20
Adjusting to the home and the company	Learning to sit still Getting into the flow of how things work in this company	16
Dealing with my supervisor	Getting direction and support Handling my supervisor's attitude and comments	11
Medications issues	Fear of distributing the wrong medications Not being able to pass medications	4
Not enough training	Didn't get any training	3
Adjusting to the field	Becoming accustomed to all the regulations	3
Paperwork	Learning how to do the paperwork	2
Issues with other jobs	Finding other jobs to supplement my income	2
The first day	The first day was a little scary.	2
Nothing was difficult	I enjoyed it all.	12
Other	Lack of privacy Getting organized	9
No response		16

$N = 1$ 38 newly hired direct support workers

Table 74. What Topics Do You Most Need Training On?

Category	Sample Responses	# of DSWs
Medication administration, psychotropics, side effects	Medication passing TMA class Side effects of medications	43
Behavioral intervention strategies	Crisis management Physical intervention Relaxation training Restraints	37
First aid, CPR	First aid CPR certification	28
Rules, regulations, and policies	Rule 40, 36 Vulnerable Adults, resident rights Policies and procedures	24
Information about specific consumers or routines	Daily living routines Consumer history	23
Implementing program plans	Program implementation Understanding consumer programs	20
Specific diagnoses	Autism Mental illness Hearing impairments	19
Specialized treatments and activities	Range of motion Safe lifting and transferring PT and OT exercises	16
Nutrition and diet	Cooking Menu planning	16
Augmentative and alternative communication	Sign language Nonverbal communication	15
Activities and community integration	Community activities and transportation Planning consumer activities	15
Computer	Computer training	12
Documentation	Paper work Specific report writing	11
Nursing procedures	Pulse and blood pressure Tube feeding Heart and lung sounds	11

Writing program plans and goals	Writing programs for consumers Writing goals	10
Seizure disorders	Seizure disorders What causes them and how to deal with them	9
Emergency procedures	Safety/emergency procedures	9
Team building Co-worker and supervisor relations	Handling conflicts with co-workers Team work Communication	8
Time and stress management	Getting enough sleep before work Priorities Stress reduction techniques	7
Career advancement	Opportunities for advancement Professionalism	6
Household maintenance	Home repair Yard work	5
Infection control	Infection control Blood-borne pathogens	5
Transporting consumers	Defensive driving	5
Finances	Handling consumer money	5
Communication	Staff and consumer interaction	4
Information about the agency/field	How the whole system works Organizational structure of this home	4
Other medical	Signs of illness Conditions and diseases Medical history and current medical status	5
Other	Supporting consumer choice Employee rights	5
None	I don't feel I need more training.	19
No response		36

N = 138 newly hired direct support workers

List Topics on Which You Most Need Training

A main task for agencies when they hire a new worker is to ensure that the worker has the knowledge, skills, and abilities to complete the job duties successfully. This study asked new workers on which topics they most needed training. The topics most frequently mentioned were medication administration, including psychotropics, and their side effects (31%), behavioral intervention strategies (27%), first aid and CPR (20%), rules, regulations, and policies (17%), and information about individual residents or routines (17%) (see Table 74).

The National Skill Standards for human services workers describes skills needed by master human service workers in 12 areas: participant empowerment, communication, assessment, community and service networking, facilitation of services, community living skills and support, education, training and self-development, advocacy, vocational, education and career support, crisis intervention, organizational participation, and documentation (Taylor, et al., 1996). The topics these new workers were most interested in training fell into either the community living skills and supports category or the crisis intervention categories on the National Skill Standards. Many National Skill Standards areas were not mentioned as priorities for training for new hires.

What Would You Tell a Friend Who Was Applying for Your Job?

The final question asked of new workers was what they would tell a best friend about this home if the friend were thinking about applying for a job (see Table 75). Workers mentioned several positive and challenging job features. Among the challenging job characteristics mentioned were challenging behavioral or medical needs (25% of workers), the need to work varying hours that included weekends and evenings (25%), and difficult or different duties such as cooking, giving medications, and providing transportation in the company vehicle (23%). The most common positive characteristics mentioned included that the job was rewarding (19%), the work environment was good (19%), you have to be responsible and mature but can have fun (17%), and you will need lots of patience (17%).

Table 75. Advice to New Employees

Category	Sample Responses	# of DSWs
Positive job features		
The job is very rewarding	It is not a glamorous job but very rewarding. It can be very fun and exciting.	26
This is a very good working environment	The company is great. Good job overall The work is enjoyable.	26
Your co-workers can be fun	The staff are excellent; lots of team work. Co-workers get along well most of the time.	23
The pay/benefits are great	The pay/benefits are great.	19
The residents are great to work with	Residents are fun. Consumers bring joy to my life.	14
The supervisor is good	Supervisors are great to work with.	11
It is an easy job	It is an easy going and self-motivating environment.	3
Neutral advice about the job		
Learn what duties are involved	Be able to cook, provide transportation Responsible for giving medications Know what is done on all shifts	32
Be responsible/mature/have fun	Use your best judgment Have a good attitude Have to work independently	24
You will need lots of patience	Be patient.	24
Treat each person with dignity and respect	Learn how to help them Understand the consumer's wants and needs. Treat them right.	20
Need to be open and flexible	Be prepared for anything. Have an open mind and remember it is just life.	15
Must enjoy working with the DD population	Make sure you know and understand the expectations of a caretaker role.	12
Training is important	Listen to orientation. Be prepared for a lot of training.	11
Ask questions	Ask specific questions about the unit. Ask about pay/benefits. Ask questions at all times.	10

Need to be compassionate and caring	It's a people job. Be caring and understanding.	10
Find the house and activity level that works for you	Spend time with the residents to see if that is where you want to be. Find a home that you like first before applying.	5

Negative job features

Resident behavior and medical needs are challenging	Consider consumer behavior problems Consumers are very medically involved. Residents can be very aggressive.	35
The hours are variable and could be difficult	Be responsible when we are short staffed. Hours are flexible. Be prepared to work weekends or evenings.	35
Pay or benefits and chances for advancement are not good	There aren't a lot of advancement opportunities. The pay isn't so great.	28
Be prepared to handle personal care for men and women	You may have to clean up after the consumers. You sometimes have to deal with things that are unappealing (urine, BM, vomit).	15
Co-workers are difficult to work with	Be discreet about your personal life. Staff backstab and lie.	14
Turnover is a problem	Expect a lot of turnover in staff. You may have to work short staffed.	12
Plan to stay	The residents need stable staff members.	12
It is a stressful job	It is mentally and emotionally demanding.	11
Some duties are physically difficult	You could be hurt on the job. It is physically hard. Need to be able to lift people.	11
There are better companies to work for	I wouldn't have them apply. Learn what the company is about/ how it is run.	7
The supervisor is bad/beware	Many staff do not like their supervisor.	5
The commute is long	It is a long way to drive.	3
Other	Are you able to leave work issues at work? Potential for layoff	6
No response/None		24

$N = 138$ newly hired direct support workers

CHAPTER 7

DISCUSSION AND RECOMMENDATIONS

This chapter begins by discussing the results of *Study 1: Facility-Level Recruitment and Retention Issues,* and *Study 2: The Study of Newly Hired Direct Support Workers,* comparing the findings of these studies with other earlier research. The second part of this chapter discusses strategies to address recruitment and retention challenges. The chapter concludes with recommendations for future research and discussion of policy implications of these studies. Limitations of these studies are also reviewed.

General Discussion

The direct support worker turnover rates in 110 small group homes for people with developmental disabilities in Minnesota, averaging 46% to 48% over 2 years, were slightly lower than the reported national averages of between 50% and 70% annually (Larson, et al., 1994). The turnover rates were much lower than the crude separation rate of 67% reported for 25 randomly selected Minnesota community residences in 1992 (Braddock & Mitchell, 1992). By contrast, in 1996 the national average turnover rate for direct support workers in public residential facilities was 18% (Larson, 1997b). National turnover rates for full-time home health aides in 1996 was estimated to be 21% (Hospital and Healthcare Compensation Service, 1996).

By the standards of virtually any industry, the turnover rates for direct support workers in the present study are very high, and they remain at levels that preclude adequately stable direct support for persons in small residential settings. In addition, many new hires were fired (15%). This termination rate remains identical to the one first reported for community residents nearly a generation ago (Lakin, 1981). Furthermore,

supervisors reported that difficulty finding new workers was their number-one agency management problem. Turnover of direct support personnel remains high and for a number of demographic, economic, and social reasons, finding new staff to replace those leaving is becoming more difficult. Clearly, recruitment and retention challenges require continuing attention and commitment by those concerned with the quality of community supports for people with developmental disabilities.

Factors Related to Recruitment and Retention Challenges

This study identified several factors that make a difference in recruitment and retention outcomes for community residential settings. One factor was the length a particular home has been in operation. For example, ICF-MR certified homes in this study, which opened much earlier than the HCBS Waiver funded homes, had significantly less turnover among direct support workers within the first 6 months of employment, had significantly higher average tenure, and hired significantly fewer new workers in a year. In addition, the average tenure of workers increased significantly overall between Time 1 and Time 2 in both types of settings. Both findings are consistent with previous studies, which identified length of operation as an important factor influencing turnover rates (e.g., Lakin, 1981).

It takes time for an agency to recruit and train a stable cadre of workers for a new home. Because the number of community residential settings nationally continues to expand rapidly (from 41,826 homes in 1992 to 78,365 homes in 1996; Prouty & Lakin, 1997), turnover challenges associated with opening new group homes and building a cadre of stable direct support workers are likely to continue. Consequently, as new small community-residential options are developed, it continues to be important to identify and implement strategies to reduce turnover, especially during the first few years of operation of a new program. For individual organizations, pacing new development may be important to avoid experiencing such "growing pains" at an agency's numerous sites. Spacing the development of new services appears particularly important in areas where unemployment is low, other job opportunities are high, and where wages and benefits in other service industries are highly competitive. This research also suggests other strategies to reduce the effects of initially high turnover rates on agencies and the people they support. These include using some established long-term employees from other sites (both supervisors and direct support workers) in new sites, increasing the proportion of positions offering full-time hours and benefits, and integrating a comprehensive program of recruitment and retention strategies into an agency's personnel practices. Elements of such comprehensive programs are identified in this monograph.

When both were measured at the same time, resident characteristics appeared to be associated with direct support worker turnover. Homes that served individuals with more extensive support needs (in level of mental retardation, challenging behavior, mental health problems, or assistance with activities of daily living) tended to have higher turnover rates. As community homes are planned for people with more substantial support needs, particular attention should be paid to factors that minimize the turnover of workers. But personnel practices that adequately support direct support workers are needed irrespective of the needs of the people they support.

The tenure of supervisors in the home is a third factor related to turnover and retention of staff. Homes that had newer supervisors

had higher turnover rates and lower average tenure than homes with more tenured supervisors (see Table 36). This is partially explained in that the maximum time a supervisor could have been in many homes was limited because many homes in the study were new (i.e., had opened within the last 5 years). However, supervisor tenure maintained its association with direct support worker turnover even after taking into consideration how long the home had been open (see Table 37). When supervisors were asked to identify factors that influenced direct support worker retention, the most commonly mentioned was supervisor turnover. In the facilities surveyed, the turnover rate for supervisors was 27% over a 12-month period.

The role of supervisors in affecting retention of direct support workers appeared very important in this study. Both staying and leaving direct support workers identified their supervisors as a key factor in leaving or wanting to leave the agency. Fair management practices were the second most common strategy identified by supervisors to address staffing problems. Direct support workers reported that having a competent supervisor was a very important expectation when they started their new jobs. Turnover rates were significantly lower in homes where the supervisors considered managing fairly to be one of their top five management practices. When supervisors were asked how the agency could help them do a better job, they requested training, improved communication, fair management practices by the agency, and support from the agency for staffing and recruitment issues. In developing interventions to address direct support worker recruitment and retention, the tenure, skills, and performance of supervisors were all important considerations.

It is, of course, impossible to overlook the importance of pay, benefits, paid leave, and promotional opportunities for the recruitment and retention of direct support workers. Not only did starting pay account for a significant portion of the variability in turnover rates at the agency level, but stayers were significantly more likely to report they thought they could get a promotion than leavers. Both direct support workers and their supervisors identified pay as a top factor influencing recruitment, retention, and plans to stay in the home. The availability of other jobs with better pay, better working conditions, or other positive conditions of employment was a significant predictor of whether direct support workers would stay or leave. Improving salaries, promotional opportunities, and benefits for direct support workers is fundamental to increasing the stability of direct support workers.

Other Findings

The relationship between direct support workers and their colleagues emerged as an important issue in the qualitative data collection. Both supervisors and direct support workers reported that team work and positive relationships among direct support workers were important to overall staff retention. Among supervisors it was tied for second among the factors viewed as influencing successful recruitment, retention, and training. Stayers identified problems with co-workers as the most common type of incident that made them want to leave. Leavers also reported that problems with co-workers had influenced their decision to leave. Several workers complained that their co-workers gossiped about them, that competition among workers in different shifts was a problem, or that poor performing co-workers made their job more difficult.

Comparisons to Other Studies

In some respects the findings of this study are consistent with those of other studies. The models of turnover presented by Arnold and Feldman (1982), Bluedorn (1982), and Michaels and Spector (1982) included all of the variables that contributed to discriminat-

ing between stayers and leavers in this study. On the other hand, a few of the variables associated with turnover in those models were not significant contributors to turnover in this study. Probably the most prominent of these is the age of the worker. Many studies have found age and turnover to be significantly related.

In this study, however, each participant was new to the agency. Once tenure was held constant, age did not predict turnover. Other studies have also reported that with age held constant statistically, only tenure predicted turnover (e.g., Porter & Steers, 1973; Zaharia & Baumeister, 1978; Lakin & Bruininks, 1981). The difference in this study is that all of the workers were new hires, so the potential confound between age and tenure was controlled through sampling rather than through statistical manipulation. This finding suggests that it is less important how old the worker is than how long the worker has been in the job when trying to predict future tenure in a specific position.

Implications and Strategies for Intervention

Many different personnel practices might be used to improve recruitment and retention of direct support workers. This section describes the implications of the study's findings for some of those strategies.

During the Application Process

Selection Strategies

Selection is the process used by organizations to improve matches between employee skills and organizational job requirements (Wanous, 1992). In this study, the 15% rate of firings for new hires by the end of 1 year indicates that improvements in selection practices could be helpful. Some improvements are quite straightforward. For example, some supervisors reported that they had to fire an employee working in the home because the employee's criminal background check came back saying the person was not eligible to work in human services. Because Minnesota state law requires this as a selection criterion and because the cost per hire for nonexempt employees in the Midwest was estimated at $2,498 and nationally was $1,388 in 1994 (JWT Specialized Communications, 1996), hiring people who will subsequently be disqualified from employment is expensive. Potential employees need to know specifically the criteria for disqualification for employment, so they do not invest their time applying for a job they will not be allowed to keep. Expedited background checks available in some states for an additional fee could reduce this problem. Additional expense could be saved by recruiting new workers in anticipation of openings so that the background checks could be completed by the time the person is needed. This strategy has the additional benefit of reducing overtime costs incurred when positions are vacant for long periods. Unfortunately, high turnover and the need to fill jobs quickly with little advance warning and with few applicants pressures supervisors to hire workers without waiting for the background checks to come in.

Structured interviews are another selection strategy that may help recruits assess their own suitability for a job and help employers assess the recruits. Structured interviews are based on a thorough job analysis that specifies critical factors in success on the job. One type of structured interview, patterned behavior description interviews, uses critical incident methodology (a strategy that asks current workers and their supervisors to describe examples of very good or very bad job performance) to identify important job dimensions and to develop a scoring guide based on examples that illustrate the range of excellent to poor performance. Then sets of questions are developed to probe the applicant's background and experience for specific examples of how that person handled situations

similar to those he or she might face in the position that is open (Wanous, 1992). Once a specific example has been identified, the interviewer probes to gather the details about the situation, how the person responded, and the outcome. Responses are scored using guidelines developed using the critical incident reporting technique. Structured interviews may be especially helpful in identifying how a recruit handles conflict with co-workers or supervisors.

It is particularly important to attend to the roles valued by direct support workers in identifying job dimensions to probe during structured interviews. Organizations tend to view jobs in terms of functional roles, but direct support workers communicated much more about the importance of the interpersonal dimensions of the role. For example, workers frequently mentioned the difficulties of adjusting to new co-workers, staff not getting along with each other, dealing with supervisors, and other interpersonal issues as one of the biggest challenges when starting the job. Study participants also identified getting along with co-workers and supervisors as an important factor in whether they would stay or leave. Asking recruits about their interpersonal responses, when there was conflict with a co-worker, can help both the employer and the potential employee to assess the likelihood that the recruit will be successful in this important aspect of direct support work.

Recruitment Sources

The pool of potential applicants for direct support work is not growing rapidly enough to provide an adequate supply of qualified applicants. Traditional recruitment practices are no longer adequate for several reasons. These reasons include: (a) demographic changes in the U.S. population indicating a decreasing number of people in the age group traditionally providing direct support workers; (b) increasing job opportunities for women outside of care-giving roles and an increasing tendency for women to accept those opportunities; (c) high unemployment rates, which create expanded job opportunities and increased wages through competition for a limited supply of job seekers; and (d) increased demand for care providers in a wide range of services for persons who are elderly or disabled. Indeed, the problem is so serious that recruitment was the number-one management problem in the homes in this study.

More effective recruitment efforts are clearly needed. Possible strategies include developing a volunteer program for students to introduce them to human services work; developing consortia of service providers in a geographic area to join together in recruitment efforts so that the field becomes more visible in the community; developing specific recruitment materials such as brochures or videotapes that could be viewed by targeted pools of potential recruits in high school and college classes, job centers, employment agencies, and community centers; and developing public service announcements.

Several states have developed preservice or in-service training and personnel preparation initiatives carried out through colleges or university programs (e.g., Kansas, New Jersey, New York, North Dakota, Wyoming), technical colleges (Minnesota), and other agencies (New Hampshire) through which new workers can be recruited (Hewitt, Larson, & Ebenstein, 1996). Other recruitment sources include paid internship programs or work study programs connected with school-to-work, welfare-to-work, or return-to-work programs.

Recruitment incentives can also be helpful. Incentive programs might pay bonuses when a new hire finishes a predetermined number of months on the job. A per-recruit-hired bonus for current workers can increase recruitment from inside sources. Incentive programs involving recruitment by current employees have the added benefit of recruiting people who were more likely to stay for at least 12 months.

Recruitment Strategies: Realistic Job Previews

Realistic job previews (RJPs) are a specific example of a broad category of strategies that many supervisors use when recruiting new workers. Realistic job previews are a refined technique to recruit people who will stay on the job and perform it with personal satisfaction because they have a "realistic" impression of the job before they accept it. Developing and instituting a realistic job preview involves: developing a good concise job description; examining turnover history in the home/agency; gathering house-specific information about the organizational climate including positive and negative job characteristics; summarizing the information; identifying a format to present the information to applicants; and implementing and evaluating the effectiveness of the RJP. The challenges for supervisors in community residential settings are to identify systematically information not already being effectively communicated, to incorporate new methods to distribute that information, and to evaluate the effectiveness of their efforts.

Characteristics of effective RJPs include:

- Make it clear to applicants that the purpose of the job preview is to help them make a thoughtful choice about whether this is a good job for them.
- Use credible information. Whenever possible use quotes from, tapes of, or results of surveys of current employees to present the information.
- Use a method to communicate the information that matches the message. Longer RJPs may work better in booklet form. Shorter RJPs may be more effective as videotapes. Make sure the videotape images match the tone of the message (negative information should not be communicated verbally by smiling workers in great surroundings). Make sure that if direct observations are used the observation of both positive and negative features of the job are included. (Meal times are a good

time for these observations in community residential settings.)

- Balance the negative and positive job factors so the RJP reflects actual negative and positive organizational characteristics experienced by the employees.
- Present the RJP information early in the application process, before the prospective employee has invested much time and effort, and before the applicant makes a commitment to the organization/job. (Wanous, 1992)

The content and quality of job previews is important. This study provided only a cursory look at the potential usefulness of RJPs. It asked supervisors to indicate how they told recruits about the job but did not delve into the content of the information provided. Studies that developed and implemented RJP interventions clearly show the benefit of the procedure in reducing turnover (e.g., Wanous, 1992; Williams, Labig, & Stone, 1993). The finding in this study that new workers with unmet expectations were more likely to leave also indicates that RJPs may be helpful. Agencies struggling with turnover and recruitment problems may benefit from examining their practices against the RJP standards listed above. In considering how to use RJPs in a particular setting, it is important to look at the following: the current ability of the organization to attract and retain newcomers; the expectations of newcomers before and after the RJP and how well those expectations reflect job realities; the ability of newcomers to select jobs that meet their job wants; initial job attitudes (satisfaction, organizational commitment, intent to stay or leave); job performance; and job survival and voluntary turnover rates (Wanous, 1992). Current employees can provide a great deal of qualitative information about aspects of employment in a specific setting that should be part of a realistic presentation of work in that setting.

This study provided information that can guide the development of RJPs. For example, direct support workers reported

that the things that made them want to stay were the people in the home (the residents and co-workers), and the rewards of being needed. Some employees found the ability to tailor hours to their needs a positive aspect of the work. Others appreciated being a valued member of a team. Among the challenging aspects of the job for some workers were physically demanding resident support needs, low pay and inadequate benefits, problems with co-workers and supervisors, and limited opportunities for advancement. Providing accurate information about these issues to recruits early in the application process is essential.

New direct support workers identified several types of information they considered important to provide to recruits. They felt positive features of the job should be stressed, such as that the job is rewarding, the residents can be fun, and the co-workers can be good and fun people. Negative features also should be addressed, including the specific nature of difficult or unpleasant tasks, specific pay and benefits' packages, and the hours the person would be expected to work. They also noted that recruits need to be fully aware of the duties and responsibilities of the job, and the need to be flexible and patient. Some of these factors are common across agencies and homes and can be included in industry-wide job preview videotapes, such as the videotape developed in Minnesota to help statewide and industry-wide recruitment efforts (Hewitt & Larson, 1996). But each agency and often each home within that agency will have specific unique job characteristics that are important to address as well, which means that more specific job preview materials are needed. Some agencies have developed their own videotapes to show potential workers the unique features of a job in those agencies.

During Organizational Entry

Orientation Strategies
The most difficult job components for new

workers in this study were becoming acquainted with the residents, learning the routines, developing relationships with co-workers, remembering training information, and adjusting to the schedule. Many expressed concern about fulfilling the substantial responsibilities given to them. The experience of entering a new organization is stressful for all workers, but is made more so when responsibility is high and direct expert support and supervision is limited as is increasingly the case in small community-service settings.

Agencies can help by communicating that the struggles facing the newcomer are typical and by providing specific suggestions about how to handle the stress they may experience. A successful orientation program will reduce the anxiety of new employees and make them feel a part of the organization; promote positive attitudes toward the job and the organization; establish open communication between the organization and the employee; communicate the expectations the organization has regarding performance and behavior; acquaint new employees with organizational background, goals, philosophies, management styles, structure, products and services; and present information on organizational policies, procedures, compensation practices, and benefits (Holland & George, 1986). Providing planned opportunities before the first solo shift for new workers to get to know other workers and the people they will be supporting can be helpful. Pacing the information provided during orientation can also help to reduce the likelihood that a new worker will become overwhelmed with the information.

Initial Socialization

Deinstitutionalization has led to widespread decentralization of services and supports. Workers who previously would have had many co-workers at the same site now may be the only worker at the site at certain times or may have only one co-worker. This shift has produced new demands, challenges, and stressors for direct support workers. It is a particular challenge to develop strategies to support workers who are in scattered sites. People need to know how to get help and to feel confident that the help they need will be available. Providing such critical information and comforts is an important part of the initial socialization process. Some agencies enhance initial socialization efforts by introducing new workers to all of the homes in a geographic area, so they always have someone to call for advice or assistance.

It is important during the initial socialization period to provide team building opportunities to help newcomers feel integrated into the social environment of the home and agency. In a study of 34 part-time workers with less than 6 months' tenure, Bachelder and Braddock (1994) found that co-worker support was significantly related to turnover in the first 6 months. Although co-worker support was not related statistically to staying or leaving among the 105 newly hired workers in this study, when staff were asked if there had been incidents that made them want to leave their jobs, the most frequent responses involved problems with co-workers. It is possible that the differences between the Bachelder and Braddock (1994) sample and the sample of new hires in this study (e.g., sample size, proportion of workers who are part time, and geographic location) account for the differences in the statistical significance of co-worker support in explaining turnover. Additional research with larger samples of new hires is probably needed to clarify this issue. In this study, stayers and leavers did not report significantly different organizational socialization practices.

Ongoing Strategies

Enhancing the Status of and Opportunities Available to Direct Support Workers

Recognizing the human needs of direct support workers to earn enough money to support themselves is fundamental to success in resolving the problems of recruiting and retaining direct support workers. It seems reasonable to assume that a major contributor to the finding that only 24% of sample members had dependents was that people with dependents find it difficult to support them on the wages and benefits available to newly hired direct support workers (only about half of new hires are eligible for benefits). Addressing the inadequacy of wages, benefits, and promotional opportunities for these workers will remain the most important issue in ensuring sustainable community services for persons with developmental disabilities.

Some efforts to enhance the status of and opportunities available to direct support workers can be made at the agency level through reorganization that flattens agency hierarchy, through restructured wage packages that offer at least prorated paid leave time (e.g., vacation) for all workers, and through flexible paid leave time and benefits policies that allow workers to use those benefits as needed in their own particular circumstances. Serious and creative thought must be given to this issue. Other efforts require systemic change. New employment benefits may be needed. Some of these could be developed in conjunction with public agencies. These might include tuition credits at public colleges, universities, and technical schools. Alternatively, tax credits can be developed to allow retirees on Social Security to benefit from employment in supporting people with disabilities. But much of the solution will also depend on increased productivity and efficiency. It will be increasingly important to consider whether certain services for some people (e.g., overnight awake support) are necessary. It will be important to look at economies that might derive from people with disabilities hiring direct support workers directly rather than through agencies. Given current financial realities with respect to public funding, attention to wages for direct support workers must focus on how current funds are spent, and how improved produc-

tivity and efficiency can be translated into wages and benefits for workers. Even with these changes, however, large-scale improvements can be made only as we see changes in public attitudes about the value of direct support workers as expressed in public policies about funding for residential services.

The status of direct support workers can be improved also by providing staff development and career advancement opportunities. In this study, stayers were significantly more likely than leavers to think promotional opportunities were available to them. Providing employee bonuses for skill development, promoting workers from within, providing educational benefits, and developing career ladders are all important to improving the stability and quality of the direct support workforce.

Staff Development for Supervisors

This study demonstrated an association between supervisor behavior and recruitment and retention outcomes. Supervisory experience was important. Homes with less tenured supervisors had significantly higher turnover rates. While this study did not specifically address factors associated with tenure for supervisors, it did suggest recruitment and training of supervisors deserves more attention than it has been given. Addressing turnover among direct support workers may well begin with success in increasing stability among their supervisors. Common practices such as rotating supervisors through settings may be detrimental to stability.

Staff development for supervisors is also important. Direct support workers identified having a good supervisor as an important issue, and reported that problems with supervision influenced their decisions to stay or leave. Supervisors themselves requested assistance. Developing training for supervisors on recruitment and retention strategies and leadership and supervision skills is important.

Ongoing Internal Evaluation Efforts

It is not sufficient for an agency to have a general idea that they have a problem with recruitment or retention. Agencies need many different types of information to monitor recruitment and retention outcomes and to design effective intervention strategies.

An Accurate Job Description. One of the first steps in designing and then evaluating an intervention strategy to better address the needs of direct support workers is to develop accurate job descriptions for all positions. Interventions such as behavioral interviewing and realistic job previews depend on having accurate up-to-date information about the jobs new workers will be expected to perform. Furthermore, initial and ongoing training depends on knowing both what information new workers need and what information master workers need to continue to grow professionally.

The information presented earlier about the skills, experiences, and needs of direct support workers and supervisors provides a starting point regarding what types of information to gather for a job analysis. Additional information is available from the Community Support Skill Standards, which describe competencies needed by master direct support workers in a variety of human services settings (Taylor, et al., 1996). The standards are based on a national job analysis.

The Community Support Skill Standards competency areas include:

- *Participant empowerment.* The competent DSW enhances the ability of the participant to lead a self-determining life by providing support and information to build self-esteem and assertiveness and to make decisions. Topics include self-determination; empowerment consumer-driven services; self-advocacy; human, legal and civil rights; decision making.

- *Communication.* The DSW should be knowledgeable about the range of effective communication and basic counseling strategies and skills necessary to establish a collaborative relationship with the participant. Topics include communication skills; augmentative and alternative communication; acronyms and terms used within the field; basic supportive counseling skills.

- *Assessment.* The DSW should be knowledgeable about formal and informal assessment practices to respond to the needs, desires, and interests of participants. Topics include assessment strategies and processes; conducting assessments; identifying preferences, capabilities, and needs of participants; using assessment tools; sharing the findings with the participant.

- *Community and service networking.* The DSW should be knowledgeable about the formal and informal supports available in his or her community and skilled in helping the participant to identify and gain access to such supports. Topics include making community connections; building support networks; identifying available community resources; outreach.

- *Facilitation of services.* The DSW should be knowledgeable about a range of participatory planning techniques and be skilled in implementing plans in a collaborative and expeditious manner. Topics include collaborative relationships; ethical standards of practice; individualized plans; strategies to achieve participant outcomes; developing successful program plans.

- *Community living and supports.* The DSW should be able to match specific supports and interventions to the unique needs of individual participants and recognize the importance of friends, family, and community relationships. Topics include human development;

sexuality; health, grooming; toileting; personal management; household management; nutrition and meal planning; laundry; transportation; adaptive equipment; physical, occupational, and communication therapy intervention; development of friendships and socialization; consumer-driven recruitment; training of service providers.

- *Education, training, and self-development*. The DSW should be able to identify areas for self-improvement, pursue needed educational or training resources, and share knowledge with others. Topics include completing required/mandated training; professional development; community outreach.
- *Advocacy.* The DSW should be knowledgeable about the diverse challenge facing participants (e.g., human rights, legal rights, administrative and financial issues) and should be able to identify and use effective advocacy strategies to overcome such challenges. Topics include identifying advocacy issues, laws, services, and community resources for people with disabilities; barriers to service delivery; negotiation.
- *Vocational, educational, and career support.* The DSW should know about the career- and education-related concerns of the participant and should be able to mobilize the resources and support necessary to help the participant to reach his or her goals. Topics include vocational assessment; opportunities for career growth and advancement; marketing skills; environmental adaptations; job interviewing; job retention; vocational services.
- *Crisis intervention*. The DSW should know about crisis intervention and resolution techniques and should match such techniques to particular circumstances and individuals. Topics include crisis intervention strategies; conflict resolution; de-escalation; environmental adaptations.

- *Organizational participation*. The DSW should be familiar with the mission and practices of the support organization and participate in the life of the organization. Topics include program evaluation; organizational structure and design; cultural sensitivity; peer support; organizational development; budgetary issues.
- *Documentation*. The DSW should be aware of the requirements for documentation in his or her organization and be able to manage these requirements efficiently. Topics include data collection and analysis; confidentiality; ethical practice; documentation strategies (Taylor, et. al., 1996).

These skill standards reflect broad competency areas important for all direct support workers. Agencies using the skill standards as a broad guide would need to identify specialized information for workers in their agencies to focus their orientation and training practices.

Retention Outcomes. Once an accurate job description has been developed, the next step in an internal evaluation of recruitment and retention outcomes is to review turnover history and establish baseline rates for the agency. Basic retention outcomes of interest include turnover rates for direct support workers and for supervisors in each site, average tenure of workers in each home, and percentage of workers who leave the home within 6 months of hire. It is also helpful to identify factors that may have contributed to the turnover rates in each home and differences in rates among homes. This includes gathering information about positive and negative job features, and describing any changes or special incentives that may have influenced retention outcomes. Establishing benchmark rates and goals for each home and for the agency as a whole allows the agency to identify homes that are struggling and those that are doing well. This can facilitate information exchanges within the agency to identify why the experiences differ across the homes. But it is also important that agency human resource personnel be reasonably sophisticated about factors associated with turnover to be able to compensate appropriately for higher rates that can be anticipated in new programs (i.e., those with high numbers of new hires), programs located in areas of low unemployment, programs in which wages compare unfavorably to prevailing wages, and so forth.

Recruitment Experiences. It is helpful for agencies to maintain information on the total number of direct support worker positions, the number of vacant positions, the number of months the longest vacancy has existed, the total cost of advertising in the previous month, and the total cost of overtime in the home for the previous month. These data observed over time can assist in monitoring organizational investments in recruitment. Parallel information should be maintained on recruitment sources and their relative effectiveness. Such an assessment could list the primary recruitment sources used by the agency (e.g., internal postings; recruitment by current employees; recruitment by former employees; paid subscription newspaper advertisements; community papers/local advertising; employment or referral agencies; temporary agencies; high school, technical colleges, or colleges; walk-ins; and other). For each source the number of applicants recruited in the last 12 months should be recorded along with the percentage of new hires from each source, the percentage of leavers from each source, and the percentage retained over different periods of time. Such information when combined with the estimated costs of each recruitment source will allow the agency to assess the relative effectiveness and cost-effectiveness of each recruitment source. Such analyses may lead agencies to invest more heavily in their most productive recruitment strategies.

Exit Interviews. Another component of an agency's self-assessment of recruitment and retention practices is an exit interview for all workers who leave their positions. This can be done by asking leavers to indicate on a scale of 1 to 5 (1 = strong reason to stay, 2 = moderate reason to stay, 3 = not a factor in my decision, 4 = moderate reason to leave, 5 = strong reason to leave) the extent to which several factors made the person want to stay or leave. Based on factors direct support workers often reported to be important in their decisions to stay or leave, items to rate could include:

- salary
- paid leave policies (sick, holiday, vacation)
- benefits policy (medical, dental, and other)
- transportation to and from work
- scheduling practices and hours worked
- opportunities for promotion or career advancement in the agency
- training and career development opportunities
- company policies regarding the treatment of people with developmental disabilities
- relationships with supervisors
- relationships with co-workers
- relationships with the people supported in the home
- specific job tasks (ask worker to specify)
- specific frustrations or disappointments (ask worker to specify)

Qualitative exit interviews are equally, if not more, useful in drawing out valuable information to assess and modify agency practices. For example, the open-ended questions in this study provided a rich source of information about the reasons direct support workers left or considered leaving their jobs. Among the most productive qualitative interview items were questions such as:

- What would you tell your best friend if he or she were considering taking your job?
- Give an example of one or two specific incidents that made you want to stay on this job.
- Give an example of one or two specific incidents that made you want to leave this job.

- What could (your supervisor/this agency) do to make your job better?
- What type of position (if any) do you plan to work after you leave this position? (e.g. direct support work elsewhere, supervisory work, job coach, a bank teller, full-time student, stay-at-home parent).

Asking leavers to respond to these questions can provide valuable information to assess and modify agency practices. Along with the specific exit interview responses, agencies will want to integrate other information including status at exit (e.g., whether leavers were fired involuntarily, left for other reasons like spousal transfer, left to complete a college degree, etc.). Agencies may also want to include the job performance of the leaver, whether the leaver will continue "on-call," and where the person went upon leaving the agency (e.g., to perform similar roles for another agency, better position in the field, lateral move for higher pay such as becoming a paraprofessional in the public schools, etc.).

Ongoing Evaluation of Current Workers. Many exit interview questions also can be asked annually of all direct support workers and first-line supervisors. Such ongoing formative evaluation allows agencies to identify and address issues as they emerge. For example, in this and other studies, organizational commitment is a predictor of whether new hires would stay or leave. Annual assessments of organizational commitment can provide an index for agencies of the current feelings of workers. Likewise regular assessments of job satisfaction could provide an indication of how workers feel about their jobs. Using such indexes over time can both identify areas of relative weakness within the organizational culture and monitor changes that might be associated with positive initiatives (e.g., a training program for supervisors) or with changing contextual factors (e.g., decreasing real dollar wages). Another area for ongoing evaluation is the extent to which the expectations of new hires were met during their first few months on the job. The results of such interviews can be used to improve the information provided to recruits before they are hired.

Recommendations for Future Research

Continued research efforts are needed to clarify recruitment and retention issues for community residential settings and emerging support models. Those efforts need to move beyond simply identifying factors associated with turnover to identifying interactions among factors, and most important, the effects of efforts to improve recruitment and retention. Among the recommendations for this future research are the following:

1. Future research on turnover should include evaluations of interventions to improve recruitment and increase retention and should clarify the conditions under which various strategies are most effective.
2. Future research should increase specificity with respect to subcategories of voluntary and involuntary turnover. For example, in this study, 16% leavers who left their regularly scheduled shifts continued to work "on-call" hours for the home.
3. Future turnover studies should include more longitudinal designs that, at minimum, measure turnover by noting whether workers *left* rather than by using proxy measures, such as intent to stay or tenure.
4. Future research in developmental disabilities' settings should include more of the emerging variables noted in personnel psychology literature, such as organizational commitment, alternative job opportunities, and met expectations, as well as variables reflecting specific realities of direct support work, such as the number of other jobs workers have and the number of hours worked at those jobs.
5. Future research should investigate recruitment and retention issues among workers who provide supports in people's own or parental homes. These developing approaches to service delivery provide

substantially different contexts for direct support work, but little is known about whether the same issues emerge or whether other issues emerge that are not evident in small group-home settings.

6. Future research should continue to investigate the impact of co-worker support and supervisory practices on turnover of new hires.

Implications for Policy

In the 9 years between June 1987 and June 1996, the number of people in the U.S. living in residential settings with six or fewer persons grew by more than 100,000 to a total of 172,540 people (Prouty & Lakin, 1997). This group now makes up a majority (53%) of the people with developmental disabilities receiving residential services outside of their family home. As more community residential settings and other community support options are developed, recruitment and retention of workers will continue to be a challenge. Public policy must play a role in responding to these challenges, even as individual supervisors, agencies, and the service provider industry as a whole accepts responsibility for their roles in responding to these challenges.

It is important to recognize the societal commitments that have been made to people with developmental disabilities. People with developmental disabilities and their family members have been taught to expect a place in their communities. These expectations are not conditioned by the ability to recruit and retain direct support workers, but recruitment and retention certainly has a tremendous impact on the extent to which these expectations can be met. In many metropolitan areas with low unemployment, requests by governmental agencies for service-providing agencies to develop new services are going unheeded, as these same agencies struggle to maintain staffing for existing services. Clearly personnel policy must become a much higher priority for all components of the develop-

mental disabilities services system, including federal, state, and local governmental agencies.

For two decades, researchers and advocates have spoken about the disgrace of paying those who support people with mental retardation wages similar to those who "wrap burgers" for a living. But this same reality continues. Today, starting wages for direct support workers average only a bit over $7.00 per hour, essentially equal to the income required to support a family of four at the federal poverty level. As a result, workers frequently work two or three jobs to support their families. Other important forms of compensation remain substandard. Almost 30% of the workers in community residential settings are not eligible for paid holiday, sick time, or vacation time. Almost 50% of the workers are not eligible for health and retirement benefits. While much can be done to improve recruitment and retention within agencies and individual homes, little of it holds much promise without wage and benefit structures for direct support workers that allow people the basic security and dignity of decent compensation for the important work they do.

Compensation must also be viewed more broadly than traditional wage and benefit packages. Providing flexible benefit packages or menus can often contribute substantially to job benefits for individuals. A worker whose health benefits are covered by a spouse's employer would view child care contributions in lieu of health insurance as a substantial increase in compensation. Companies that individually or jointly with other agencies provide high-quality child care, particularly for people working nontraditional hours such as evenings, weekends, and holidays, frequently provide a benefit that money cannot buy and without which many people simply cannot consider direct support work. Companies that offer transportation to employees to get to work may provide a benefit that translates into "compensation" by removing or reducing the cost of owning a vehicle, and, for persons working nighttime hours, may provide compensation in terms of added security.

In addition to creative uses of existing compensation resources, new forms of compensation need to be sought. State legislatures that find it difficult to increase direct funding allocations to increase resources for compensation need to be challenged to support significant alternative benefits such as tuition credits for public colleges and universities based on hours worked, free or discounted admissions to state parks, and other direct benefits. They also need to be asked to attend to meaning-ful regulatory reform that assures that people with disabilities have the protections and professional services they need while assuring that the maximum appropriate amounts of allocated resources are given to the direct support workers who provide those protections and services.

In addition to adequate compensation for their work, workers must sense a future in their work if they are to be retained. By its very nature, direct support work will appeal to people in transitional periods of their lives (e.g., college students or people needing part-time or nontraditional work schedules). These people often bring vitality, creativity, and other positive attributes to the work setting. But stability in the worksite depends on a stable cadre of experienced skilled workers who see a positive future in their work. Such perceptions depend on career ladders and training structures that develop, recognize, and reward valued skills. Such structures need to be unbounded by individual agencies to permit and promote advancement opportunities through movement to new employers and new roles. Development of high-quality supervisory training programs is particularly important, both for advancement opportunities afforded, and because of the clear impor-

tance of supervisory skills in developing and sustaining the direct support workforce.

Coinvolvement of government is also needed in expanding the pool of persons familiar with and able to consider direct support work. It is no longer enough to view personnel recruitment strictly as the problem of individual agencies. Governmen-tal entities need to invest in materials (e.g., videotapes, brochures), activities (e.g., provoding booths at job fairs, making public service announcements, developing school-to-work curricula), and opportunities (e.g., welfare-to-work training funds) which contribute to expanding the pool of potential direct support workers.

Welfare-to-work is an example of an area in which state and local government can work with the service provider industries to respond to the challenges of labor shortages in direct support work. Designating direct support work as a target industry for welfare-to-work efforts would provide jobs for people who need them and provide support for people who need help.

Commitments to direct support work opportunities for welfare recipients entering the workforce make good use of the system's existing entry-level training, flexible hours, and supportive work environments; the work is readily available in almost all communi-ties. Indeed, creative welfare-to-work models train people in their own neighborhoods or in local community centers or schools to provide support for persons with disabilities in those same communities. Of course there are challenges, but many of these challenges are interrelated with personnel problems. For example, child care is frequently needed by people leaving welfare to go to work. Because many direct support workers' schedules include evening, night, weekend, and holiday work, finding adequate child care is even more difficult. Some human service agencies have begun to address this issue by individu-ally or collectively providing company-sponsored child care for their workers. Such worker supports not only contribute to an ability to participate in welfare-to-work initiatives, but they also increase viability of direct support work for new pools of potential employees and help sustain current employees.

The number and stability of direct support workers can also be increased by finding ways to offer cost-effective benefits. This may require changing policies that prevent agencies from developing joint purchasing agreements for health care. Such arrangements could reduce the cost of health care for workers by providing a bigger pool of people to be insured. Because many agencies are small (providing supports in an average of 20 homes), such joint purchasing could provide substantial cost savings that could be reinvested into salaries and paid leave to reduce turnover rates.

This society has made a clear commitment to the presence and participation of people with developmental disabilities in its communities, schools, and work places. That commitment is in jeopardy. Demographic shifts depleting the numbers of young adults, economic growth resulting in more available jobs, increasing wages, and human service expansion, and other factors are making it increasingly difficult to maintain current levels of staff much less to expand the number of staff available to meet future needs. A crisis in the community flows from what has been inadequate attention to the intractable connection between community living for people with disabilities and community supports provided by direct support workers.

Of course aspects of the crisis will be self-correcting. The economic boom of 1998 inevitably will end. The numbers of young adults will increase early in the next decade. But even if it were possible to ride out these most difficult years, there are compelling reasons not to do so. Economic downturns may create a greater supply of potential employees, but it will also create

greater demand for their services and greater demand for resources to finance them. On the other end of the demographic "baby boomlet" that will bring more young adults into the workplace in the next decade is a population of persons aged 85 years and older that is projected to grow 56% between 1995 and 2010. This group will increase the demand for direct supports and services. In short, the problems of recruiting and retaining direct support workers will continue to demand concerted and creative efforts by public officials, advocates, service providers, and others who care about the well-being of persons with developmental disabilities. Areas of particular focus include increased amounts and attractive options in compensation, more comprehensive and more effective recruitment initiatives, improved quality, recognition of and transferability of training, expanded career opportunities, more effective supervision, better matching of employees to work roles, and more effective team building. Success in these efforts is important to assuring that community living is a real and viable option for all Americans with developmental disabilities.

We must not encourage the respect and dignity of one group of people (those with developmental disabilities) at the expense of another group of people (those paid to support them). Americans talk often of the importance of having good teachers for our children. We value those who would help children to become productive citizens of this nation. We must also respect those who help and support people with mental retardation and other developmental disabilities.

Study Limitations

There are several limitations to this study. One limitation resulted from its longitudinal nature. Both supervisors and direct support workers were asked to complete multiple surveys. The response rates for the surveys varied. The direct support worker exit questionnaires, in particular, were completed by only a small portion of all study participants. Response rate problems occurred because of the repeated number of surveys required, because both supervisors and direct support workers left the home or the agency during the study, and because of the length of the surveys. Several supervisors and direct support workers dropped out of the study because of its demands. This problem was minimized in this analysis by focusing heavily on the first facility survey, and the first two direct support worker surveys.

Attrition of direct support workers was anticipated in the study design. Attrition among supervisors meant that for homes in the study, each time a new supervisor was added, the new supervisor had to be asked if he or she would consent to participate. A few homes were dropped from the study when a new supervisor declined to continue participation. Despite these difficulties, more than 87% of supervisors and direct support workers completed all of the surveys necessary for this monograph.

A related limitation is that the participation rate for new hires in this study was somewhat lower than desired. Supervisors often reported that a new hire quit after orientation or after a few days on the job, and supervisors were not able to enroll that person in the study before he or she left. Fully one third of the workers asked to participate chose not to do so. The impact of not including these workers is unknown. It is possible that workers most likely to leave in the first few weeks of employment chose not to participate in the study because they knew they would not be staying very long.

Another potential limitation was the sensitivity of the study questions. Two strategies were used to minimize this problem. First, a group of potential respondents was consulted during the development of the instruments to make the questions as clear, relevant, and nonthreatening as possible. Second, the surveys were returned in sealed envelopes with assurances to the respondents of complete confidentiality. This strategy seemed to work as supervisors and direct support workers readily reported sensitive information such as the firing of a study participant or problems with supervisors and co-workers. Confidentiality was further promised and provided by limiting information available from the study to aggregate results.

Another limitation was that half of the homes in the study were not randomly selected. Fifty-four (of 110) homes were selected because they were part of another study of people moving out of one of Minnesota's Regional Treatment Centers. On the other hand, 56 of the 110 homes were randomly selected to participate in this study. Altogether, 83 of 188 residential service provider agencies in Minnesota participated. Despite its limitations, this study is the most comprehensive examination of personnel outcomes in community residential settings in Minnesota and is one of the largest longitudinal studies of direct support workers in homes supporting six or fewer people in the nation.

REFERENCES

Abelson, M. A., & Baysinger, B. D. (1984). Optimal and dysfunctional turnover: Toward an organizational level model. *Academy of Management Review, 9*, 331-341.

Allen, N. J., & Meyer, J. P. (1990). Organizational socialization tactics: A longitudinal analysis of links to newcomers' commitment and role orientation. *Academy of Management Journal, 33*, 847-858.

Alpha Group. (1990). *Report to the commissioner of the Minnesota Department of Human Services by the task force on the compensation and training of direct care employees.* St. Paul: Minnesota Department of Human Services Task Force on Compensation and Training of Direct Care Staff.

American Association of University Affiliated Programs for Persons. (1996). *Community services training initiatives.* Silver Springs, MD: Author.

Arnold, H. J., & Feldman, D. C. (1982). A multi-variate analysis of the determinants of job turnover. *Journal of Applied Psychology, 67*, 350-360.

Askvig, B. A., & Vassiliou, D. (1991). *Factors related to staff longevity and turnover in a facility serving persons with developmental disabilities.* Minot: Minot State University, North Dakota Center for Disabilities.

Bachelder, L., & Braddock, D. (1994). *Socialization practices and staff turnover in community homes for people with developmental disabilities.* Chicago: University of Illinois at Chicago, Institute on Disability and Human Development, College of Associated Health Professions.

Balfour, D. L. & Neff, D. M. (1993). Predicting and managing turnover in human service agencies: A case study of an organization in crisis. *Public Personnel Management, 22*, 473-486.

Bass, A. R., & Agar, J. (1991). Correcting point-biserial turnover correlations for comparative analysis. *Journal of Applied Psychology, 76*, 595-598.

Baumeister, A. A., & Zaharia, E. S. (1987). Withdrawal and commitment of basic-care staff in residential programs. In S. Landesman & P. Vietz (Eds.). *Living environments and mental retardation* (pp. 229-267). Washington, DC: American Association on Mental Retardation.

Baysinger, B. D., & Mobley, W. M. (1983). Employee turnover: Individual and organizational analysis. *Research in Personnel and Human Resources Management, 1*, 269-319.

Bennett, N., Blum, T. C., Long, R. G, & Roman, P. M. (1993). A firm-level analysis of employee attrition. *Group and Organizational Management, 18*, 482-499.

Bluedorn, A. C. (1982). The theories of turnover: Causes, effects, and meaning. *Research in the Sociology of Organizations, 1*, 75-128.

Borofsky, G. L., Bielema, M., & Hoffman, J. (1993). Accidents, turnover, and use of a preemployment screening inventory. *Psychological Reports, 73*, 1067-1076.

Braddock, D., & Mitchell, D. (1992). *Residential services for persons with developmental disabilities in the United States: A national study of staff compensation, turnover, and related issues.* Washington, DC: American Association on Mental Retardation.

Breaugh, J. A. (1983). Realistic job previews: A critical appraisal and future research directions. *Academy of Management Review, 8*, 612-619.

Bruininks, R. H., Kudla, M. J., Wieck, C. A., & Hauber, F. A. (1980). Management problems in community residential facilities. *Mental Retardation, 18*, 125-130.

Bycio, P., Hackett, R. D., & Alvares, K. M. (1990). Job performance and turnover: A review and meta-analysis. *Applied Psychology: An International Review, 39,* 47-76.

Camp, R. R., Blanchard, N. P., & Huszczo, G. E. (1986). *Toward a more organizationally effective training structure and practice.* Engelwood Cliffs, NJ: Prentice Hall.

Campion, M. A. (1991). Meaning and measurement of turnover: Comparison of alternative measures and recommendations for research. *Journal of Applied Psychology, 76,* 199- 212.

Cardona, S. M., & Bernreuter, M. (1996). Graduate nurse overhires: A cost analysis. *Journal of Nursing Administration, 26,* 10-15.

Carston, J. M., & Spector, P. E. (1987). Unemployment, job satisfaction, and employee turnover: A meta-analytic test of the Muchinsky model. *Journal of Applied Psychology, 72,* 374-381.

Cohen, A. (1993). Organizational commitment and turnover: A meta-analysis. *Academy of Management Journal, 36,* 1140-1157.

Colbert, J. A., & Wolff, D. E. (1992). Surviving in urban schools: A collaborative model for a beginning teacher support system. *Journal of Teacher Education, 43,* 193-199.

Coleman, T. E., & Craig, C. (1981). *The community personnel study: Turnover issues in mental retardation community programs.* Boston, MA: Massachusetts Department of Mental Health, Division of Mental Retardation.

College of Administrative Science. (1957). *Leader Behavior Description Questionnaire.* Columbus: Ohio State University.

Cotton, J. L., & Tuttle, J. M. (1986). Employee turnover: A meta-analysis and review with implications for research. *Academy of Management Review, 11,* 55-70.

Covert, S. B. (1995). *Listening to New Hampshire's caregivers: Conference proceedings.* Concord: New Hampshire Developmental Disabilities Council.

Dalton, D. R., & Todor, W. D. (1982). Turnover: A lucrative hard dollar phenomenon. *Academy of Management Review, 7,* 212-218.

Dalton, D. R., Todor, W. D., & Krackhardt, D. M. (1982). Turnover overstated: The functional taxonomy. *Academy of Management Review, 7,* 117-123.

Department of Employee Relations. (1989). *Study of employee wages, benefits, and turnover in Minnesota direct care facilities serving persons with developmental disabilities.* St. Paul: State of Minnesota, Department of Employee Relations for the Department of Human Services.

Ditson, L. A. (1994). Efforts to reduce homemaker/home health aide turnover in a home care agency. *Journal of Home Health Care Practices, 6,* 33-44.

Dunnette, M. D., Arvey, R. D., & Banas, P. A. (1973). Why do they leave? *Personnel, 50* (3), 25-39.

Ebenstein, W., & Gooler, L. (1993). *Cultural diversity and developmental disabilities workforce issues: A report on the developmental disabilities workforce in New York City.* New York: Consortium for the Study of Disabilities, City University of New York.

Feldman, P. H. (1993). Work life improvements for home care workers: Impact and feasibility. *Gerontologist, 33,* 47-54.

Ferris, K. R. & Aranya, N. (1983). A comparison of two organizational commitment scales. *Personnel Psychology, 36,* 87-98.

Fiorelli, J. S., Margolis, H., Heverly, M. A., Rothchild, E., & Krasting, D. J. III. (1982). Training resident advisors to provide community residential services: A university-based program. *Journal of The Association for Persons With Severe Handicaps, 7,* 13- 19.

Gaddy, T., & Bechtel, G. A. (1995). Nonlicensed employee turnover in a long-term care facility. *Health Care Supervision, 13*, 54-60.

Ganju, V. (1979). *Turnover trends among MHMR series employees in Texas state schools.* Austin: Texas Department of Mental Health and Mental Retardation.

George, M. J., & Baumeister, A. A. (1981). Employee withdrawal and job satisfaction in community residential facilities for mentally retarded persons. *American Journal of Mental Deficiency, 85*, 639-647.

Governor's Planning Council on Developmental Disabilities. (1992). *Minnesotans speak out: A summary of town meetings held throughout Minnesota on developmental disabilities issues.* St. Paul: Author.

Griffin, R. W., & Bateman, T. S. (1986). Job satisfaction and organizational commitment. In C. L. Cooper & I. Robertson (Eds.). *International Review of Industrial and Organizational Psychology* (pp. 157-188). New York: John Wiley & Sons.

Hafdahl, R. P. (1995). *ARRM wage and benefit survey: Direct care staff in private community residential servcies serving people with developmental disabilities.* St. Paul: Association for Residential Resources in Minnesota.

Halpin, A. W. (1957). *Manual for the Leader Behavior Description Questionnaire.* Columbus: Ohio State University, College of Commerce and Administration.

Hatton, C., & Emerson, E. (1993). Organizational predictors of staff stress, satisfaction, and intended turnover in a service for people with multiple disabilities. *Mental Retardation, 31*, 388-395.

Hayden, M. F., DePaepe, P., Soulen, T. & Polister, B. (1995). *Deinstitutionalization and community integration of adults with mental retardation: Summary and comparison of the baseline and one-year follow-up residential data for the Minnesota Longitudinal Study.* Minneapolis: Research and Training Center on Residental Services and Community Living, University of Minnesota.

Hayden, M. F., Soulen, T., Schleien, S. J., & Tabourne, C. E. S. (1996). A matched, comparative study of the recreation integration of adults with mental retardation who moved into the community and those who remained at the institution. *Therapeutic Recreation Journal, 30*, 41-63.

Hewitt, A., & Larson, S. A. (1995). *Turnover and training in community residential settings: A statewide comparison across service types and job functions.* Minneapolis: Research and Training Center on Residential Services and Community Living, University of Minnesota. Unpublished manuscript.

Hewitt, A., & Larson, S. A. (Executive Producers). (1996). *Helping hand: An introductory video on a career in direct service.* Minneapolis: Institute on Community Integration; St. Cloud, MN: St. Cloud Technical College.

Hewitt, A., & Larson, S. A. (Eds.). (1997). *Personnel Initiative '97: A comprehensive workforce development plan for human services workers.* St. Paul: Alliance for Consumer Options.

Hewitt, A., Larson, S. A., & Ebenstein, W. (1996). State initiatives to address direct support worker issues. In T. Jaskulski, & W. Ebenstein (Eds.). *Opportunities for excellence: Supporting the frontline workforce* (pp. 19-39). Washington, DC: President's Committee on Mental Retardation.

Hewitt, A., Larson, S. A., Ebenstein, W., & Rose, J. (1996). Future directions: Creating a sufficient, competent and stable direct support workforce for the 21st Century. In T. Jaskulski, & W. Ebenstein (Eds.). *Opportunities for excellence: Supporting the frontline workforce* (pp.120-137). Washington, DC: President's Committee on Mental Retardation.

Hewitt, A., Larson, S. A., & O'Nell, S. (1996). National voluntary credentialling for direct service workers. *Policy Research Brief, 8* (2). Minneapolis: University of Minnesota, Institute on Community Integration.

Hewitt, A., O'Nell, S., & Larson, S. A. (1996). Overview of direct support workforce issues. In T. Jaskulski, & W. Ebenstein (Eds.). *Opportunities for excellence: Supporting the frontline workforce* (pp. 1-18). Washington, DC: President's Committee on Mental Retardation.

Hill, B. K., Lakin, K. C., Bruininks, R. H., Amado, A. N., Anderson, D. J., & Copher, J. I. (1989). *Living in the community: A comparative study of foster homes and small group homes for people with mental retardation.* Minneapolis: University of Minnesota, Center for Residential and Community Services.

Holland, J. E., & George, B. W. (1986). Orientation of new employees. In J. J. Famularo (Ed.). *Handbook of human resources administration* (2nd ed.) (pp.1-24, 35). New York: McGraw-Hill.

Hom, P. W., & Griffeth, R. W. (1991). Structural equations modeling test of a turnover theory: Cross-sectional and longitudinal analyses. *Journal of Applied Psychology, 76,* 350-366.

Hom, P. W., Griffeth, R. W., & Sellaro, C. L. (1984). The validity of Mobley's (1977) model of employee turnover. *Organizational Behavior and Human Performance, 34,* 141- 174.

Hom, P. W., Caranikas-Walker, F., Prussia, G. E., & Griffeth, R. W. (1992). A meta-analytic structural equations analysis of a model of employee turnover. *Journal of Applied Psychology, 77,* 890-909.

Hospital and Healthcare Compensation Service. (1996). *Home care salary and benefits report, 1996-1997.* Oakland, NJ: Author.

Huselid, M. A. (1995). The impact of human resource management practices on turnover, productivity, and corporate financial performance. *Academy of Management Journal, 38,* 635-672.

Huselid, M. A., & Day, N. E. (1991). Organizational commitment, job involvement, and turnover: A substantive and methodological analysis. *Journal of Applied Psychology, 76,* 380-391.

Irvine, D. M., & Evans, M. G. (1995). Job satisfaction and turnover among nurses: Integrating research findings across studies. *Nursing Research, 44,* 246-253.

Jackofsky, E. F. (1984). Turnover and job performance: An integrated process model. *Academy of Management Review, 9,* 74-83.

Jackofsky, E. F., & Peters, L. H. (1983). Job turnover versus company turnover: Reassessment of the March and Simon Participation Hypothesis. *Journal of Applied Psychology, 68,* 490-495.

Jacobson, J. W., & Ackerman, L. J. (1989). *Staff attitudes and the group home as a work place.* Albany: New York State Office of Mental Retardation and Developmental Disabilities.

Jacobson, J. W., & Ackerman, L. J. (1992). Factors associated with staff tenure in group homes serving people with developmental disabilities. *Adult Residential Care Journal, 6,* 45-60.

Jaskulski, T., & Metzler, C. (1990). *Forging a new era: The 1990 reports on people with developmental disabilities, Appendix.* Washington, DC: National Association of Developmental Disabilities Councils.

Jaskulski, T., & Whiteman, M. (1996). Family member perspectives on direct support workers. In T. Jaskulski, & W. Ebenstein (Eds.). *Opportunities for excellence: Supporting the frontline workforce* (pp. 56-75). Washington, DC: President's Committee on Mental Retardation.

Jones, A. A., Blunden, R., Coles, E., Evens, G., & Porterfield, J. (1981). Evaluating the impact of training, supervision, feedback, self-monitoring, and collaborative goal setting on staff and client behavior. In J. Hogg & P. Mittler (Eds.). *Staff training in mental handicap* (pp. 213-299). Cambridge, MA: The MIT Press.

Jones, G. R. (1986). Socialization tactics, self-efficacy, and newcomers' adjustments to organizations. *Academy of Management Journal*, *29*, 262-279.

JWT Specialized Communications. (1996). *Cost per hire statistics*. Figures based on reports from the Employment Management Association. Http://www.jwtworks.com.

Kemery, E. R., Dunlap, W. P., & Bedeian, A. G. (1989). Criterion specification in employee separation research: Tenure or turnover? *Best papers proceedings* (pp. 387-391). Columbia, SC: Academy of Management.

Kirkbride, F. B. (1912). The institution as a factor in race conservation. In T. M. Mulry (Chair). *Third New York City conference on charities and corrections* (pp. 141-151). Albany, NY: J. B. Lyon.

Kline, C. J., & Peters, L. H. (1991). Behavioral commitment and tenure of new employees: A replication and extension. *Academy of Management Journal*, *34*, 194-204.

Knight, C. B., & Hayden M. F. (1989). *Workforce 2000: Will our communities be able to meet the needs of Wisconsin's citizens with developmental disabilities*. Madison: Wisconsin Council on Developmental Disabilities Community Direct Service Worker Taskforce.

Lakin, K. C. (1988). Strategies for promoting the stability of direct care staff. In M. P. Janicki, M. W. Krauss, & M. M. Seltzer (Eds.). *Community residences for persons with developmental disabilities* (pp. 231-238). Baltimore: Paul H. Brookes.

Lakin, K. C. (1981). *Occupational stability of direct-care staff of residential facilities for mentally retarded people*. Doctoral dissertation. Minneapolis: University of Minnesota.

Lakin, K. C., Blake, E. M., Prouty, R. W., & Mangan, T. (1993). *Residential services for persons with developmental disabilities: Current status and trends through 1991*. Minneapolis: Center on Residential Services and Community Living, University of Minnesota.

Lakin, K. C., & Bruininks, R. H. (1981). *Occupational stability of direct-care staff of residential facilities for mentally retarded people*. Minneapolis: University of Minnesota, Department of Psychoeducational Studies, Center for Residential Services and Community Living.

Lakin, K. C., Hill, B. K., Chen, T. H., & Stephens, S. A. (1989). *Persons with mental retardation and related conditions in mental retardation facilities: Selected findings from the 1987 National Medical Expenditure Survey*. Minneapolis: University of Minnesota, Center for Residential Services and Community Living.

Lakin, K. C., & Larson, S. A. (1992). Satisfaction and stability of direct care personnel in community-based residential services. In J. W. Jacobson, S. N. Burchard & P. J. Carling (Eds.) *Community living for people with developmental and psychiatric disabilities* (pp. 244-262). Baltimore: Johns Hopkins University Press.

Larson, S. A. (1997). [Staffing patterns and outcomes in public residential facilities 1996 by state]. Unpublished raw data.

Larson, S. A., Hewitt, A., & Anderson, L. (In Press). Staff recruitment challenges and interventions in agencies supporting people with developmental disabilities. *Mental Retardation*.

Larson, S. A., Hewitt, A., & Lakin, K. C. (1994). Residential services personnel: Recruitment, training and retention. In M. Hayden & B. Abery (Eds.). *Challenges for a service system in transition: Ensuring quality community experiences for persons with developmental disabilities* (pp. 313-341). Baltimore: Paul H. Brookes.

Larson, S. A., & Lakin, K. C. (1991). Parent attitudes about residential placement before and after deinstitutionalization: A research synthesis. *Journal of The Association for Persons With Severe Handicaps, 16*, 25-38.

Larson, S. A., & Lakin, K. C. (1992). Direct-care staff stability in a national sample of small group homes. *Mental Retardation, 30*, 13-22.

Larson, S. A., & Lakin, K. C. (1995). *Status and changes in Medicaid's Intermediate Care Facility for the Mentally Retarded (ICF-MR) program: Results from anaylsis of the Online Survey Certification and Reporting System*. Minneapolis: University of Minnesota, Research and Training Center on Residential Services and Community Living.

Leftwich, K. (1994). Job outlook 2005: Where to find the good jobs. *Vocational Education Journal, 6*, 27-29.

Legislative Budget and Finance Committee. (1989). *Report on salary levels and their impact on quality of care for client contact workers in community-based MH/MR and child care programs*. Harrisburg: Pennsylvania General Assembly.

Levy, P. H., Levy, J. M., Freeman, S., Feiman, J., & Samowitz, P. (1988). Training and managing residences for persons with developmental disabilities. In M. P. Janicki, M. W. Krauss, & M. M. Seltzer (Eds.). *Community residences for persons with developmental disabilities* (pp. 239-249). Baltimore: Paul H. Brookes.

Louis, M. R. (1980). Surprise and sense making: What newcomers experience in entering unfamiliar organizational settings. *Administrative Science Quarterly, 25*, 226-251.

Louis, M. R., Posner, B. Z., & Powell, G. N. (1983). The availability and helpfulness of socialization practices. *Personnel Psychology, 36*, 857-866.

Major, D. A., Kozlowski, S. W. J., Chao, G. T., & Gardner, P. D. (1995). A longitudinal investigation of newcomer expectations, early socialization outcomes, and the moderating effects of role development factors. *Journal of Applied Psychology, 80*, 418-431.

Mathieu, J. E., & Zajac, D. M. (1990). A review and meta-analysis of the antecedents, correlates, and consequences of organizational commitment. *Psychological Bulletin, 108*, 171-194.

McDonnell, W. A., & Wilson-Simpson, D. (1994). Atmosphere assessment in residential treatment. *Residential Treatment for Children & Youth, 12*, 25-37.

McEvoy, G. M., & Cascio, W. F. (1985). Strategies for reducing employee turnover: A meta-analysis. *Journal of Applied Psychology, 70*, 342-353.

McEvoy, G. M., & Cascio, W. F. (1987). Do good or poor performers leave? A meta-analysis of the relationship between performance and turnover. *Academy of Management Journal, 30*, 744-762.

Meglino, B. M., DeNisi, A. S., & Ravlin, E. C. (1993). Effects of previous job exposure and subsequent job status on the functioning of a realistic job preview. *Personnel Psychology, 46*, 803-822.

Meglino, B. M., DeNisi, A. S., Youngblood, S. A., & Williams, K. J. (1988). Effects of realistic job previews: A comparison using an enhancement and a reduction preview. *Journal of Applied Psychology, 73*, 259-266.

Michaels, C. E., & Spector, P. E. (1982). Causes of employee turnover: A test of the Mobley, Griffeth, Hand, and Meglino model. *Journal of Applied Psychology, 67,* 53-59.

Minnesota State Technical College Task Force on Educational Opportunities for Developmental Disabilities Service Providers (1993). *State Technical College Task Force on Educational Opportunities for Developmental Disabilities Service Providers.* St. Paul: Minnesota Technical College System.

Mitra, A., Jenkins, G. D., & Gupta, N. (1992). A meta-analytic review of the relationship between absence and turnover. *Journal of Applied Psychology, 77,* 879-889.

Mobley, W. H. (1982). *Employee turnover: Causes, consequences, and control.* Reading, MA: Addison-Wesley.

Mobley, W. H., Griffeth, R. W., Hand, H. H., & Meglino, B. M. (1979). Review and conceptual analysis of the employee turnover process. *Psychological Bulletin, 86,* 493-522.

Mobley, W. H., Horner, S. O., & Hollingsworth, A. T. (1978). An evaluation of precursors of hospital employee turnover. *Journal of Applied Psychology, 63,* 408-414.

Morrison, E. W. (1993). Longitudinal study of the effects of information seeking on newcomer socialization. *Journal of Applied Psychology, 78,* 173-183.

Mowday, R. T., Porter, L. W., & Steers, R. M. (1982). *Employee-organization linkages: The psychology of commitment, absenteeism, and turnover.* New York: Academic Press.

Mowday, R. T., Steers, R. M., & Porter, L. W. (1979). The measurement of organizational commitment. *Journal of Vocational Behavior, 14,* 224-247.

Muchinsky, P. M., & Morrow, P.C. (1980). A multi-disciplinary model of voluntary employee turnover. *Journal of Vocational Behavior, 17,* 263-290.

Mueller, C. W., & Price, J. L. (1989). Some consequences of turnover: A work unit analysis. *Human Relations, 42,* 389-402.

Orcutt, C. (1989). *A review of the staffing situation of the direct care workers in the developmental disabilities field.* Salem: State of Oregon, Executive Department, Budget and Management Division.

Ostroff, C., & Kozlowski, S. W. J. (1992). Organizational socialization as a learning process: The role of information acquisition. *Personnel Psychology, 45,* 849-874.

Ostroff, C., & Kozlowski, S. W. J. (1993). The role of mentoring in the information gathering process of newcomers during early organizational socialization. *Journal of Vocational Behavior, 42,* 170-183.

Pierson, J. (1993). *Impact of organizational factors on employee turnover in agencies serving people with developmental disabilities.* Baltimore: Maryland State Planning Council on Developmental Disabilities.

Porter, L. W., & Steers, R. M. (1973). Organizational, work, and personal factors in employee turnover and absenteeism. *Psychological Bulletin, 80,* 151-176.

Premack, S. L., & Wanous, J. P. (1985). A meta-analysis of realistic job preview experiments. *Journal of Applied Psychology, 70,* 706-719.

Price, J. L. (1977). *The study of turnover.* Ames: Iowa State University Press.

Price, J. L. (1989). The impact of turnover on the organization. *Work and Occupations, 16,* 461-473.

Price, J. L., & Mueller, C. W. (1986). *Absenteeism and turnover of hospital employees.* Greenwich, CT: JAI Press.

Prouty, R., & Lakin, K. C. (1997). *Residential services for persons with developmental disabilities: Status and trends through 1996.* Minneapolis: University of Minnesota, Center for Residential Services and Community Living.

Randall, D. M. (1990). The consequences of organizational commitment: Methodological investigation. *Journal of Organizational Behavior, 11,* 361-378.

Razza, N. J. (1993). Determinants of direct-care staff turnover in group homes for individuals with mental retardation, *Mental Retardation, 31,* 284-291.

Rice, R. W., Peirce, R. S., Moyer, R. P., & McFarlin, D. B. (1991). Using discrepancies to predict the perceived quality of work life. *Journal of Business and Psychology, 6,* 39- 55.

Rusbult, C. E., Farrell, D., Rogers, G., & Mainous, A. G. III. (1988). Impact of exchange variables on exit, voice, loyalty, and neglect: An integrative model of responses to declining job satisfaction. *Academy of Management Journal, 31,* 599-627.

Saks, A. M. (1994). A psychological process investigation for the effects of recruitment source and organization information on job survival. *Journal of Organizational Behavior, 15,* 225-244.

Smith, P., Schiller, M. R., Grant, H. K., & Sachs, L. (1995). Recruitment and retention strategies used by occupational therapy directors in acute care, rehabilitation, and long-term care settings. *American Journal of Occupational Therapy, 49,* 412-419.

Staw, B. M. (1980). The consequences of turnover. *Journal of Occupational Behaviour, 1,* 253-273.

Steel, R. P., & Griffeth, R. W. (1989). The elusive relationship between perceived employment opportunity and turnover behavior: A methodological or conceptual artifact? *Journal of Applied Psychology, 74,* 846-854.

Steel, R. P., & Ovalle, N. K. II (1984). A review and meta-analysis of research on the relationship between behavioral intentions and employee turnover. *Journal of Applied Psychology, 69,* 673-686.

Steel, R. P., Shane, G. S., & Griffeth, R. W. (1990). Correcting turnover statistics for comparative analysis. *Academy of Management Journal, 33,* 179-187.

Steers, R. M., & Mowday, R. T. (1981). Employee turnover and post-decision accommodation processes. *Research in Organizational Behavior, 3,* 235-281.

Stumpf, S. A., & Hartman, K. (1984). Individual exploration to organizational commitment or withdrawal. *Academy of Management Journal, 27,* 308-329.

Sullivan, T. G. (1982). Organizational commitment, job satisfaction, and leadership behaviors within residential facilities for the mentally retarded (Doctoral dissertation, University of Pittsburgh). *Dissertations Abstracts International,* No. 8303641.

Task Force on Human Resources Development. (1989). *Human resources in community human service programs: Report to the Secretaries of Aging, Health, and Public Welfare.* Harrisburg, PA: Author.

Taylor, G. S. (1994). The relationship between sources of new employees and attitudes toward the job. *Journal of Social Psychology, 134,* 99-110.

Taylor, M., Bradley, V., & Warren, R., Jr., (1996). *The community support skill standards: Tools for managing change and achieving outcomes.* Cambridge, MA: Human Services Research Institute.

Tett, R. P., & Meyer, J. P. (1993). Job satisfaction, organizational commitment, turnover intention, and turnover: Path analyses based on meta-analytic findings. *Personnel Psychology, 46,* 259-293.

U.S. Bureau of the Census. (1996). *Statistical abstract of the United States: 1996* (116th ed.). Washington, DC: U.S. Government Printing Office.

Van Maanen, J., & Schein, E.H. (1979). Toward a theory of organizational socialization. *Research in Organizational Behavior, 1,* 209-264.

Wanous, J. P. (1989). Installing a realistic job preview: Ten tough choices. *Personnel Psychology, 42,* 117-134.

Wanous, J. P. (1992). *Organizational entry: Recruitment, selection, orientation and socialization of newcomers* (2nd ed.). New York: Addison Wesley.

Wanous, J. P., Poland, T. D., Premack, S. L., & Dawis, K. S. (1992). The effects of met expectations on newcomer attitudes and behaviors: A review and meta-analysis. *Journal of Applied Psychology, 77,* 288-297.

Wanous, J. P., Stumpf, S. A., & Bedrosian, H. (1979). Job survival of new employees. *Personnel Psychology, 32,* 651-662.

Weiss, D. J., Dawis, R B., England, G. W., & Lofquist, L. J. (1967). *Manual for the Minnesota Satisfaction Questionnaire.* Minneapolis: University of Minnesota, Vocational Psychology Research.

Whiteman, M., & Jaskulski, T. (1996). Consumer perspectives on direct support workers. In T. Jaskulski, & W. Ebenstein (eds.). *Opportunities for excellence: Supporting the frontline workforce* (pp. 40-55). Washington, DC: President's Committee on Mental Retardation.

Williams, C. R., Labig, C. E., & Stone, T. H. (1993). Recruitment sources and posthire outcomes for job applicants and new hires: A test of two hypotheses. *Journal of Applied Psychology, 78,* 163-172.

Williams, C. R., & Livingstone, L. P. (1994). Another look at the relationship between performance and voluntary turnover. *Academy of Management Journal, 37,* 269-298.

Zaharia, E. S., & Baumeister, A. A. (1978). Technician turnover and absenteeism in public residential facilities. *American Journal of Mental Deficiency, 82,* 580-593.

Zaharia, E. S. & Baumeister, A. A. (1981). Job preview effects during the critical initial employment period. *Journal of Applied Psychology, 66,* 19-22.

APPENDIX A
FACILITY SURVEYS

FACILITY SURVEY—Time 1

Date: _____   Facility ID: _____

Supervisor Name: _____   Facility Name: _____

Supervisor Title: _____   Agency ID: _____

Telephone Number: _____   Agency Name: _____

Instructions: This survey should be completed by the on-site supervisor responsible for hiring, firing, training and providing direct supervision to new direct service staff members in this home. Please answer each question as accurately as possible. If you do not understand a question, answer it as well as you can and write a note in the margin explaining your question. If there are questions that you cannot answer, please ask the person in your agency who has the answer or provide that person's name and phone number so we can contact them. *Your answers to these questions will be kept confidential and will not be shared with your employer.* **If you have questions or need more information, please call Sherri Larson at 612-624-6024.**

A. Supervisor Characteristics

1. Gender (mark one)
   - _____ 0. male
   - _____ 1. female

2. How old are you?
   - _____ 1. 15-25 years
   - _____ 2. 26-35 years
   - _____ 3. 36-45 years
   - _____ 4. 46-55 years
   - _____ 5. 56-65 years
   - _____ 6. 66-75 years
   - _____ 7. 76-85 years

3. How many years of paid employment experience do you have working with people with developmental disabilities?
   - _____ years

4. How long have you worked in this home?
   - _____ years _____ months

5. How many years of school have you finished? (circle one number)
   - 9 (Junior High School)
   - 10
   - 11
   - 12 (High school graduate or GED)
   - 13
   - 14 (Associate or 2 year degree)
   - 15
   - 16 (Four year degree)
   - 17
   - 18 (Master's level degree)
   - 19
   - 20
   - 21 (Doctoral degree)

6. How many hours per week (on average) do you spend working *at this home*?

  _____ number of hours

7. How many people in each category do you now directly supervise at this home?

  _____ a. direct service staff members

  _____ b. supervisors

  _____ c. professional support staff

  _____ d. non-professional support staff

8. How many different program sites are you currently responsible for?

  _____ number of homes/facilities

B. Facility Characteristics

1. What is the <u>total</u> dollar amount your agency receives <u>per day</u> to provide services to <u>all</u> of the people living in this home? (including room and board - if applicable)

  $ _____ total per day

2. How many people with developmental disabilities live in this home?

  _____ number of people

3. What year did *this home* begin providing residential services to persons with developmental disabilities?

  19_____

4. Which of the following licensing or certification categories best describes the services provided in this home? (Mark one)

  _____ 1. Federal Intermediate Care Facilities/Mental Retardation (ICF-MR)

  _____ 2. Medicaid Home and Community Based Waiver

_____ 3. Semi-independent Living Services (SILS)

_____ 4. Adult Foster Care (not waiver or SILS)

_____ 5. Other

5. How many different residential sites does your agency operate in Minnesota?

  _____ # of different sites

6. What type of agency operates this home? (Mark one)

  _____ 1. state operated (SOCS)

  _____ 2. county operated

  _____ 3. corporate profit

  _____ 4. corporate non-profit

  _____ 6. family (not incorporated)

7. What year did *your agency* begin providing services to persons with developmental disabilities?

  19_____

8. Are the direct service staff members in this home part of a union? (mark one)

  _____ 0. no

  _____ 1. yes

  8a. If yes, how long have these employees been unionized?

  _____ years _____ months

9. What city/municipality is this home located in (If in a metropolitan area, be specific - for example, if the home is in Bloomington, do not write Minneapolis)?

  _____

10. What county is this home located in?

  _____

138

C. Characteristics of the Direct Service Staff Members

Direct service staff members are people whose primary job responsibility is to provide support, training, supervision and personal assistance to people with developmental disabilities in this home.

1. On average, how many direct service staff members are on duty at the following times (including those who may be on break)?

Weekdays	Weekends
_____ a. 7:30 am	_____ e. 7:30 am
_____ b. 3:00 pm	_____ f. 3:00 pm
_____ c. 7:30 pm	_____ g. 7:30 pm
_____ d. 2:00 am	_____ h. 2:00 am

2. Counting all shifts (if applicable) and weekends, how many <u>different</u> direct service staff members, including part-time, work specific regular shifts in this home?

_____ number direct service staff who work regular shifts in this home

3. How many *different* direct service staff members, including part-time, work in this home *only* on an "on call" or emergency basis?

_____ number of direct service staff who work *only* "on call" hours in this home

4. How many different people (including part- time) provide direct supervision or management services for direct service staff members in this home?

_____ number of different people

5. Do any paid direct service staff members live at this address? (mark one)

_____ 0. no

_____ 1. yes

6. Counting all shifts (if applicable) and weekends, how many direct service staff members, including part-time persons (not including "on call" staff), left their direct service staff position for any reason during the last 12 months?

_____ a. total who left a direct service position in this home for any reason in the last 12 months

_____ b. number who had worked in this home for less than 6 months

_____ c. number who had worked in this home for 6 to 12 months

_____ d. number who had worked in this home over 12 months

7. Which of the following professionals provide services *at this location* to one or more persons living in this home? (Mark all that apply)

_____ a. Nurse (RN or LPN)

_____ b. Nutritionist/dietician

_____ c. Physical Therapist (PT or PTA)

_____ d. Speech/Language or Communication Therapist

_____ e. Occupational Therapist (OT or COTA)

_____ f. Social Worker (non-county)

_____ g. Recreation Therapist

_____ h. Psychiatrist

_____ i. Psychologist

_____ j. Behavior Analyst or Consultant

_____ k. Audiologist

_____ l. Advocate

_____ m. Other _____

8. Which of the following non-professional support services are provided to this home by people *other than* direct service staff members? (Mark all that apply)

_____ a.   cook

_____ b.   gardener/lawn maintenance

_____ c.   cleaning person

_____ d.   maintenance/repair person

_____ e.   drivers

_____ f.   laundry

_____ g.   other _____

9. Which of the following tasks are performed by direct service staff members alone or with the assistance of the people living in this home? (check all that apply)

_____ a.   prepare meals

_____ b.   gardening/lawn maintenance

_____ c.   cleaning

_____ d.   building maintenance/repair

_____ e.   provide transportation for residents

_____ f.   laundry

_____ g.   set up program plans/meetings

_____ h.   attend program planning meetings

_____ i.   write program plans

_____ j.   supervise other staff or schedule shifts

_____ k.   hire replacements

_____ l.   other _____

10. How many direct service staff members from this home were promoted to supervisory or management positions in your agency in the last 12 months? (These supervisory or management positions may require some direct care.)

_____ number of people

11. How many direct service staff members from this home moved from part-time to full-time positions with this agency during the last 12 months?

_____ number of people

12. Please indicate the current beginning and maximum wage for direct service staff members now working in this home.

Awake staff

a. $_____/hr beginning wage (low)

b. $_____/hr current maximum wage

Sleep night staff

e. $_____/hr beginning wage (low)

f. $_____/hr current maximum wage

13. What factors are considered when setting a wage for a new direct service staff member? (mark all that apply)

_____ a.   educational background

_____ b.   experience in the field

_____ c.   job title

_____ d.   number of hours worked per week

_____ e.   other _____

14. Under what conditions do direct service staff members in this home earn a salary differential (higher pay)? (mark all that apply)

_____ a.   overnight shifts

_____ b.   weekend hours

_____ c.   evening hours

_____ d.   holidays

_____ e.   over 40 hours in one week/80 hours in two weeks

_____ f.   full-time status

_____ g.   other _____

5. What factors influence whether a direct service staff member will get a permanent salary increase? (mark all that apply)

_____ a. number of months worked

_____ b. performance review

_____ c. increase in the number of hours worked per week

_____ d. increased job responsibilities

_____ e. promotion to another direct service position

_____ f. changes in union contracts

_____ g. other

16. How many hours per week must a direct service employee work to be considered *full-time* by your agency?

_____ number of hours per week

17. How many hours per week must a *part-time* employee work to be eligible for paid leave time (e.g., sick, holiday or personal leave) from your agency?

_____ number of hours per week

18. How many hours per week must a *part-time* employee work to be eligible for benefits (e.g., health insurance) from your agency?

_____ number of hours per week

19. Does your agency have a probationary period for newly hired direct service staff members? (mark one)

_____ 0. no

_____ 1. yes

19a. If yes, how many months does the probationary period last?

_____ months

20. Please indicate the maximum amount of paid leave time (in days per year) that *direct service staff members* can earn:

Paid Leave	Full-time Number of days per year				Part-time (50% time workers) Number of days per year			
	Upon hire	After probation	After 1 year	After 5 years	Upon hire	After probation	After 1 year	After 5 years
Sick								
Vacation								
Holiday								
Personal Leave								
Other _____								

21. Using the scale (0-3) below, please indicate which benefits are offered to *direct service staff*:

0 = benefit not offered
1 = benefit offered, employee covers total cost
2 = benefit offered, agency covers part cost
3 = benefit offered, agency covers total cost

Benefit	Full-time	Part-time
Health insurance (self)		
Health insurance (dependent)		
Dental plan (self)		
Dental plan (dependent)		
Life insurance (self)		
Retirement plan (other than social security)		
Child care		
Tuition		
Other		

D. Recruitment and Retention Experiences

1. Do you have problems finding new direct service staff members? (mark one)

_____ 0. no

_____ 1. yes

2. Approximately how many applicants did you have the last time you hired a direct service staff member to work a weekend position in this home?

_____ number of applicants

3. The last time you hired a direct service staff member to work a weekend position, how many people did you extend a job offer to before the person who actually started working was hired (including the person who took the job)?

_____ # people offered the position

4. How satisfied were you that the last person you hired in a direct service staff position would fulfill the job requirements for that position? (mark one)

_____ 1. very satisfied

_____ 2. satisfied

_____ 3. somewhat satisfied

_____ 4. somewhat dissatisfied

_____ 5. dissatisfied

_____ 6. very dissatisfied

5. What are the primary limitations (if any) of recent applicants for direct service positions? (Mark all that apply)

_____ a. None

_____ b. Lack of specific training

_____ c. Lack of basic communication skills (written, spoken)

     d.   Lack of experience with people with developmental disabilities

     e.   Lack of experience with job responsibilities

     f.   Lack of maturity (e.g., experience managing a household, money management skills)

     g.   other _____

. How much difficulty is caused by the amount of staff turnover in this home? (mark one)

     1.   very much

     2.   much

     3.   little

     4.   very little or none

. When do new direct service staff members first see a copy of their job description? (mark one)

     1.   when they get the application

     2.   when they return the application

     3.   after applying, before being hired

     4.   after being hired, before starting work

     5.   the first day of work

     6.   during the probationary period

     7.   after the probationary period

     8.   never

8. **Realistic job previews** tell applicants what to expect in a job, including features of the job that the person may not expect and may not like (e.g., having to work holidays, or working with persons who may injure them). This information is presented <u>before</u> the applicant decides to take the job. Does your agency use realistic job previews when hiring direct service staff members? (mark one)

     0.   no

     1.   yes

8a.   If your agency uses realistic job previews which of the following types of information are provided before a job is offered? (mark all that apply)

     a.   none (we do not use realistic job previews)

     b.   written information

     c.   audio or video information

     d.   verbal descriptions

     e.   direct observation of people in the home

     f.   other

9.   Which of the following tasks do you handle for direct service staff members in this home? (mark all that apply)

     a.   advertising job openings

     b.   responding to inquiries about openings

     c.   screening applications

     d.   interviewing applicants

     e.   hiring new employees

     f.   agency orientation

     g.   house orientation

     h.   ongoing training

     i.   performance evaluation

     j.   firing employees

     k.   other _____

10. Please provide the following information for each *direct service staff member currently* employed in this home (not including "on call" staff).

Employee	Age (in years) 1 = 15-25 years 2 = 26-35 years 3 = 36-45 years 4 = 46-55 years 5 = 56-65 years 6 = 66-75 years 7 = 76-85 years	Gender 0 = male 1 = female	Hours worked per week at this home	Number of months worked in this home (round up for partial months)
01				
02				
03				
04				
05				
06				
07				
08				
09				
10				
11				
12				
13				
14				
15				
16				
17				
18				
19				
20				
21				
22				

1. Agency Management Practices and Problems

1. Which of the following are the major problems in operating and maintaining your facility? (check all that apply)

____ a. Admissions policies
____ b. Community attitude toward residents
____ c. Certification and licensing
____ d. Developing individualized program plans
____ e. Difficulty finding qualified staff
____ f. Difficulty maintaining sufficient average daily resident population
____ g. Funding mechanism problems (e.g., late checks, county control)
____ h. Government regulations
____ i. Inadequate funds
____ j. Insurance problems
____ k. Lack of advocacy services
____ l. Lack of alternative community residential placements
____ m. Lack of community support services
____ n. Lack of coordination between provider agencies
____ o. Lack of follow-along services
____ p. Lack of program implementation
____ q. Lack of comprehensive state planning
____ r. Maintenance, physical plant, capital expenditures
____ s. Need for transportation services
____ t. Problems with residents
____ u. Problems with family members
____ v. Quality assurance
____ w. Relationships with board of directors
____ x. Staffing patterns and work conditions
____ y. Staff motivation
____ z. Staff training and development
____ aa. Staff turnover
____ bb. Start-up money and costs
____ cc. Unions/Labor relations
____ dd. Wage and hour considerations
____ ee. Workman's compensation
____ ff. Other _____

2. Which five of the following management practices are the most effective strategies your agency uses to address staffing issues for direct service staff members. (check five items from the list)

____ a. Communicate clear, understandable program objectives, and agency philosophy
____ b. Communicate the importance of each staff member to the agency
____ c. Encourage team work among staff
____ d. Encourage social involvement among employees
____ e. Establish effective communication among staff
____ f. Hire specific types of people/ask new hires for a time commitment.
____ g. Manage in a way that is perceived by staff to be fair
____ h. Provide a mechanism for complaints to management
____ i. Provide competitive pay and benefits
____ j. Provide employee fitness and wellness programs
____ k. Provide employee autonomy in their jobs, encourage creativity
____ l. Provide realistic information about the job to applicants.
____ m. Provide staff recognition
____ n. Support the staff members
____ o. Train supervisors to provide effective supervision to increase staff satisfaction with supervision
____ p. Treat staff fairly
____ q. Use a participatory management structure
____ r. Use a decentralized management structure - limit agency hierarchy
____ s. Use clear and understandable job roles and responsibilities
____ t. Other _____

F. Characteristics of the people living in this home. Please provide updated information about the people living in this home. The responses provided for last year's survey are enclosed for your reference.

Characteristic	1	2	3	4	5	6	7	8	9	10	11	12	13	14	15
Age (in years) 1 = 0-10 yrs, 2 = 11-20, 3 = 21-30, 4 = 31-40, 5 = 41-50, 6 = 51-60, 7 = 61-70, 8 = 71-80, 9 = 81-90															
Level of Mental Retardation 1 = normal (IQ 86+), 2 = borderline (IQ 71-85), 3 = mild (IQ 56-70), 4 = moderate (IQ 41-55), 5 = severe (IQ 26-40), 6 = profound (IQ 25 or less)															
Gender (0 = male, 1 = female)															
Year moved to this home 19___															
Moved here from a reg. treatment center (0 = no, 1 = yes)															
Autism (0 = no, 1 = yes)															
Blind or uncorrected vision impairment (0 = no, 1 = yes)															
Brain or neurological damage (0 = no, 1 = yes)															
Cerebral palsy (0 = no, 1 = yes)															
Deaf or uncorrected hearing impairment (0 = no, 1 = yes)															
Current epilepsy or seizure disorder (0 = no, 1 = yes)															
Mental illness - formal diagnosis (0 = no, 1 = yes)															
Specific planned intervention for challengingbehavior (e.g., aggression or self-injurious behavior) (0 = no, 1 = yes)															
Walks without assistance (0 = no, 1 = yes)															
Dresses without assistance (0 = no, 1 = yes)															
Eats without assistance (0 = no, 1 = yes)															
Independent in toileting (less than 1 day-time accident per month) (0 = no, 1 = yes)															
Communicates by talking (0 = no, 1 = yes)															

Thank you for your help.

Minnesota Study of Newly Hired Residential Direct Service Staff Members
FACILITY SURVEY—Time 2

Date: _____   Facility ID: _____

Supervisor Name: _____   Facility Name: _____

Supervisor Title: _____   Agency ID: _____

Telephone Number: _____   Agency Name: _____

Instructions: This survey should be completed by the on-site supervisor in this home. Please answer each question as accurately as possible. If you do not understand a question, answer it as well as you can and write a note in the margin explaining your question. If there are questions that you cannot answer, please ask the person in your agency who has the answer or provide that person's name and phone number so we can contact them. *Your answers to these questions will be kept confidential and will not be shared with your employer.* **If you have questions or need more information, please call Sherri Larson at 612-624-6024.**

A. Supervisor Characteristics

1. Gender (mark one)

    _____ 0.   male

    _____ 1.   female

2. How old are you?

    _____ 1.   15-25 years

    _____ 2.   26-35 years

    _____ 3.   36-45 years

    _____ 4.   46-55 years

    _____ 5.   56-65 years

    _____ 6.   66-75 years

    _____ 7.   76-85 years

3. How many years of paid employment experience do you have working with people with developmental disabilities?

    _____ years

4. How long have you worked for this agency?

    _____ years _____ months

5. How long have you worked in this home?

    _____ years _____ months

6. How many years of school have you finished? (circle one number)

    9 (Junior High School)

    10

    11

    12 (High school graduate or GED)

    13

    14 (Associate or 2 year degree)

    15

    16 (Four year degree)

    17

    18 (Master's level degree)

    19

    20

    21 (Doctoral degree)

7. Did you take any courses on mental retardation or on working with people who have disabilities as part of your general education (e.g., in college)? (mark one)

_____ 0. no

_____ 1. yes

8. Are you currently enrolled in vocational/ technical school, college, or graduate school? (mark one)

_____ 0. no

_____ 1. yes

  8a. If yes, do you intend to continue working in your present position when you have completed your education? (mark one)

_____ 0. no

_____ 1. yes

9. How many hours per week (on average) do you spend working at this home in each of the following roles? (Please provide a single number rather than a rang of numbers.)

_____ a. number of hours per week working direct care

_____ b. number of hours per week in supervisory or paper work roles

10. Did you fill out the Time 1 Facility Survey for the *Minnesota Direct Service Staff Study* (mark one)?

_____ 0. no

_____ 1. yes

11. Are you the on-site supervisor for this house (mark one)?

_____ 0. no

_____ 1. yes

12. How many different program sites do you currently supervise?

_____ number of homes/facilities

13. How many people in each category do you now directly supervise at this home?

_____ a. direct service staff members

_____ b. supervisors

_____ c. professional support staff

_____ d. non-professional support staff

14. Which of the following tasks do you handle regarding direct service staff members in this home? (mark all that apply)

_____ a. advertising job openings

_____ b. responding to inquiries about openings

_____ c. screening applications

_____ d. interviewing applicants

_____ e. hiring new employees

_____ f. agency orientation

_____ g. house orientation

_____ h. ongoing training

_____ i. performance evaluation

_____ j. firing employees

_____ k. other _____

B. Facility Characteristics

1. Which of these licensure categories best describes this home? (mark one)

_____ 1. Intermediate Care Facility-Mental Retardation (ICF-MR, Rule 34)

_____ 2. Supervised Living Services (SLS - Rule 42)

_____ 3. Semi-Independent Living Services (SILS - Rule 18)

_____ 4. Other_____

2. What is the *total* dollar amount your agency receives *per day* to provide services to *all* of the people living in this home? (including room and board - if applicable)

$ _____ total per day

3. How many people with developmental disabilities live in this home?

_____ number of people

4. What is the zip code for this home?

_____

5. What county is this home located in?

_____

6. In what city/municipality is this home located? (If in a metropolitan area, be specific - for example, if the home is in Bloomington, do not write Minneapolis.)

_____

C. Characteristics of the Direct Service Staff Members

Direct service staff members are people whose primary responsibility is to provide support, training, supervision and personal assistance to people with developmental disabilities in this home.

1. On average, how many direct service staff members are on duty at the following times (including those who may be on break)?

Weekdays		Weekends	
_____	a. 7:30 am	_____	e. 7:30 am
_____	b. 3:00 pm	_____	f. 3:00 pm
_____	c. 7:30 pm	_____	g. 7:30 pm
_____	d. 2:00 am	_____	h. 2:00 am

2. Counting all shifts (if applicable) and weekends, how many <u>different</u> direct service staff members, including part-time, work specific regular shifts in this home?

_____ number of direct service staff who work regular shifts in this home

3. How many *different* direct service staff members, including part-time, work in this home *only* on an "on call" or emergency basis?

_____ number of direct service staff who work only "on call" hours in this home

4. How many different people (including part- time) provide direct supervision or management services for direct service staff members in this home?

_____ number of different people

5. Do any paid direct service staff members live at this address? (mark one)

_____ 0. no

_____ 1. yes

6. How many new direct service staff members did you approach about participating in this study?

_____ a. num. who agreed to participate and carried through

_____ b. num. who agreed to participate but did not carry through

_____ c. num. who decided not to participate

7. Which of the following professionals provide services *at this location* to one or more persons living in this home? (mark all that apply)

_____ a. Nurse (RN or LPN)

_____ b. Nutritionist/dietician

_____ c. Physical Therapist (PT or PTA)

_____ d. Speech/Language or Communication Therapist

_____ e. Occupational Therapist (OT or COTA)

_____ f. Social Worker (non-county)

_____ g. Recreation Therapist

_____ h. Psychiatrist

_____ i. Psychologist

_____ j. Behavior Analyst or Consultant

_____ k. Audiologist

_____ l. Advocate

_____ m. Other _____

8. Which of the following non-professional support services are provided to this home by people *other than* direct service staff members? (mark all that apply)

_____ a. cook

_____ b. gardener/lawn maintenance

_____ c. cleaning person

_____ d. maintenance/repair person

_____ e. drivers

_____ f. laundry

_____ g. other

9. Which of the following tasks are performed by direct service staff members alone or with the assistance of the people living in this home? (mark all that apply)

_____ a. prepare meals

_____ b. gardening/lawn maintenance

_____ c. cleaning

_____ d. building maintenance/repair

_____ e. provide transportation for residents

_____ f. laundry

_____ g. set up program plans/meetings

_____ h. attend program planning meetings

_____ i. write program plans

_____ j. supervise other staff or schedule shifts

_____ k. hire replacements

_____ l. other _____

10. What is the *current* beginning and maximum wage for direct service staff members now working in this home?

Awake staff

a. $ _____/hr beginning wage (lowest)

b. $ _____ /hr current maximum wage

Sleep night staff

c. $ _____/hr beginning wage (lowest)

d. $ _____/hr current maximum wage

e. _____N/A sleep night staff not used

11. Has the union status of direct service staff members in this home changed during the last 12 months? (mark one)

_____ 0. no

_____ 1. yes - a union was voted in

_____ 2. yes - a union was voted out

12. Has your agency changed its policies regarding paid leave time (e.g., personal leave, sick, holiday, vacation) during the last 12 months? (mark one)

_____ 0. no

_____ 1. yes

12a. If yes, how has the paid leave time policy been changed? (mark all that apply)

_____ a. increased number of hours of paid leave time

_____ b. decreased number of hours of paid leave time

_____ c. increase number of employees eligible for paid leave time

_____ d. decreased number of employees eligible for paid leave time

_____ e. modified the types of paid leave offered (e.g., personal leave)

_____ f. other _____

13. Has your agency changed its policies regarding benefits (e.g., health care, dental) during the last 12 months? (mark one)

_____ 0. no

_____ 1. yes

13a. If yes, how has the benefits policy been changed? (mark all that apply)

_____ a. increased agency contribution toward employee coverage for existing benefits

_____ b. decreased agency contribution toward employee coverage for existing benefits

_____ c. increased number of employees eligible for benefits

_____ d. decreased number of employees eligible for benefits

_____ e. added specific types of benefits (e.g., health care, dental plan, tuition)

_____ f. eliminated specific types of benefits

_____ g. added or increased agency contribution for dependents

_____ h. eliminated or decreased agency contribution for dependents

_____ f. other _____

14. Please provide the following information for each *direct service staff member currently* employed in this home (not including "on call" staff). A copy of the Time 1 chart for this home has been included for your reference.

Employee	Age (in years) 1 = 15-25 years 2 = 26-35 years 3 = 36-45 years 4 = 46-55 years 5 = 56-65 years 6 = 66-75 years 7 = 76-85 years	Gender 0 = male 1 = female	Hours worked per week at this home	Number of months worked in this home (round up for partial months)
01				
02				
03				
04				
05				
06				
07				
08				
09				
10				
11				
12				
13				
14				
15				
16				
17				
18				
19				
20				
21				
22				

D. Recruitment Experiences

1. Do you have problems finding new direct service staff members? (mark one)

    _____ 0. no

    _____ 1. yes

2. Approximately how many applicants did you have the last time you hired a direct service staff member to work a weekend position in this home?

    _____ number of applicants

3. The last time you hired a direct service staff member to work a weekend position, how many people did you extend a job offer to before the person who actually started working was hired (including the person who took the job)?

    _____ number of people offered the position

4. How satisfied were you that the last person you hired in a direct service staff position would fulfill the job requirements for that position? (mark one)

    _____ 1. very satisfied

    _____ 2. satisfied

    _____ 3. somewhat satisfied

    _____ 4. somewhat dissatisfied

    _____ 5. dissatisfied

    _____ 6. very dissatisfied

5. Do employees in your agency receive any formal incentives for recruiting new direct service staff members to work for your agency (mark one)

    _____ 0. no

    _____ 1. yes - financial incentive only

    _____ 2. yes - other type of incentive only (e.g., paid time off)

    _____ 3. yes - both financial and other types of incentives

6. What are the primary limitations (if any) of recent applicants for direct service positions? (mark all that apply)

    _____ a. none

    _____ b. lack of specific training

    _____ c. lack of basic communication skills (written, spoken)

    _____ d. lack of experience with people with developmental disabilities

    _____ e. lack of experience with job responsibilities

    _____ f. lack of maturity (e.g., experience managing a household, money management skills)

    _____ g. other

7. How useful are each of the following strategies in recruiting new direct service staff members to work in this home (rate each item)?

    3 = Very helpful
    2 = Somewhat helpful
    1 = Not helpful
    0 = Not used

    _____ a. internal postings

    _____ b. recruitment by current/ former employees

    _____ c. newspaper advertisements

    _____ d. tv or radio advertisements

    _____ e. employment/referral agency

    _____ f. high school, technical college, or college placement office/job board

    _____ g. other _____

8. When do new direct service staff members first see a copy of their job description? (mark one)

_____ 1. when they get the application

_____ 2. when they return the application

_____ 3. after applying, before being hired

_____ 4. after being hired, before starting work

_____ 5. the first day of work

_____ 6. during the probationary period

_____ 7. after the probationary period

_____ 8. never

9. **Realistic job previews** tell applicants what to expect in a job, including features of the job that the person may not expect and may not like (e.g., having to work holidays, or working with persons who may injure them). This information is presented *before* the applicant decides to take the job. Does your agency use realistic job previews when hiring direct service staff members? (mark one)

_____ 0. no

_____ 1. yes

9a. If your agency uses realistic job previews which of the following strategies are used to provide information to applicants before a job is offered? (mark all that apply)

_____ a. none (we do not use realistic job previews)

_____ b. written information

_____ c. audio or video information

_____ d. verbal descriptions

_____ e. direct observation of people in the home

_____ f. other _____

154

E. Retention and Turnover Experiences

1. Counting all shifts including weekends, how many *direct service staff members*, including part-time persons (not including "on call" staff), left their direct service staff position for any reason during the last 12 months?

_____ Total who left a direct service position in this home in the last 12 months

1a. For the direct service staff members who left in the last 12 months, how long had they worked at this home before leaving?

_____ a. number who left after less than 6 months

_____ b. number who left after 6 to 12 months

_____ c. number who left after more than 12 months

2. How much difficulty is caused by the amount of staff turnover in this home? (mark one)

_____ 1. very much

_____ 2. much

_____ 3. little

_____ 4. very little or none

3. How many direct service staff members from this home were promoted to supervisory or management positions in your agency in the last 12 months? (These supervisory or management positions may require some direct care.)

_____ number of people

4. How many new/returning/transferring direct service staff members have been hired to work regularly scheduled shifts at this house during the last 12 months (Include persons who actually were paid

for one or more hours of work. Do not include persons hired only to work temporary, on-call or fill-in hours).

_____ number of different people

5. How many direct service staff members from this home moved from part-time to full-time positions with this agency during the last 12 months?

_____ number of people

6. How many different people have worked in the role of on-site supervisor at this house in the last 12 months (count yourself if you are an on-site supervisor)?

_____ number of different people

7. Do you use a temporary agency to provide direct service staff for this house?

_____ 0. no

_____ 1. yes

If yes,

7a. What company do you use?
_____

7b. How many shifts did temporary agency staff work at this house in the last 30 days?

_____ number of shifts

7c. How satisfied are you with the services of the temporary agency?

_____ 1. very satisfied

_____ 2. satisfied

_____ 3. dissatisfied

_____ 4. very dissatisfied

F. Training Experiences and Issues

1. Which of the following are major difficulties for this home in training direct service staff members? (mark all that apply)

____ a. Finding financial resources to pay trainers or consultants, purchase materials, and/or to pay registration costs.

____ b. Finding resources to staff homes while direct service staff members are participating in training activities

____ c. Finding qualified trainers within the company to address training needs

____ d. Finding qualified trainers from outside the company to address specific training needs

____ e. Finding conferences, courses or workshops that address the most important training needs for direct service staff members

____ f. Finding conferences, courses or workshops close enough to the home

____ g. Finding conferences, courses or workshops that are reasonably priced

____ h. Finding high quality training materials

____ i. Getting accurate, timely information about training opportunities

____ j. Arranging training at times when direct service staff members can attend

____ k. Planning training for staff members with widely differing experiences and knowledge

____ l. Providing training that actually results in changes in staff job performance

____ m. Providing timely high quality training to newly hired direct service staff members

____ n. Finding incentives to motivate staff to get training

____ o. Finding resources to retain staff once they have completed training

____ p. Other _____

2.. The following skills have been identified as important for persons who supervise direct service staff in residential programs. For each skill please use the following scale to indicate how much <u>you</u> currently know about the topic (rate each item).

4 = I know the topic well enough to provide advanced training to other supervisors.
3 = I know a lot about the topic but could benefit from advanced training.
2 = I know about the topic but could benefit from basic training.
1 = I know little about this topic and could benefit from a basic introduction and comprehensive training.

Area 1: Providing leadership and management of staff

____ 1.1 Supervise staff providing direct care

____ 1.2 Demonstrate working knowledge of individual habilitation programs

____ 1.3 Delegate duties to other staff

____ 1.4 Establish and modify staff work schedules

____ 1.5 Utilize and coordinate activities of specialized service staff

____ 1.6 Supervise volunteers

____ 1.7 Plan and conduct staff meetings

____ 1.8 Provide periodic individual supervisory feedback for staff support, education, and accountability

____ 1.9 Conduct formal periodic staff evaluations

____ 1.10 Provide staff counseling and referrals for additional services

____ 1.11 Ensure adequate staff development, education and training

____ 1.12 Build effective work teams

____ 1.13 Create a positive work environment

____ 1.14 Encourage staff participation in decisions

____ 1.15 Make decisions based on analysis of individual situations, needs and issues

____ 1.16 Assist in interviewing/hiring new employees

____ 1.17 Operate in accordance with agency policy, philosophy and goals

____ 1.18 Fulfill supervisory responsibilities in a labor/management setting

____ 1.19 Assist management in planning, developing and disseminating programs

____ 1.20 Maintain ongoing communication with next-level management and others outside the work unit

____ 1.21 Assist your supervisor to carry out assigned responsibilities

Area 2: Ensuring quality and integration of services

____ 2.1 Function as a member of the treatment team

____ 2.2 Supervise active treatment and implementation of individual treatment plans

____ 2.3 Establish staff work schedule in coordination with activity schedules of person receiving services

____ 2.4 Ensure daily documentation of progress toward individual program goals

____ 2.5 Demonstrate appropriate intervention skills in working with persons receiving services

____ 2.6 Assist in coordination of services between program area and residence

156

____ 2.7 Ensure that required health care practices are followed

____ 2.8 Support recreation staff in coordinating recreational programming

____ 2.9 Maintain a humanistic program environment for persons receiving services

____ 2.10 Supervise protection of individual rights

Area 3: Developing and maintaining operational systems

____ 3.1 Supervise maintenance of a safe and clean environment

____ 3.2 Conduct inspections of work unit

____ 3.3 Maintain security of program resources and personal items

____ 3.4 Supervise implementation of emergency procedures in accordance with agency policy

____ 3.5 Coordinate and ensure incident reporting

____ 3.6 Take preliminary steps in an investigation of an incident

____ 3.7 Ensure proper food handling and storage techniques

____ 3.8 Ensure that individuals receive prescribed diets

____ 3.9 Coordinate availability of transportation resources

____ 3.10 Maintain financial systems for the work unit

____ 3.11 Coordinate purchasing and/or ordering of equipment and supplies

____ 3.12 Ensure that all required reports are completed

____ 3.13 Maintain program coordination

____ 3.14 Establish and maintain local practices for work unit

Area 4: Developing and maintaining community relations

____ 4.1 Establish and maintain community relations

____ 4.2 Establish and maintain positive relations with families and friends of individuals receiving services

____ 4.3 Assist in establishing community contacts to facilitate integration and normalization

____ 4.4 Educate the community regarding persons with MR/DD

____ 4.5 Access community resources

Area 5: Ensuring standards compliance

____ 5.1 Review and monitor program activities for standards compliance

____ 5.2 Communicate and share program information with staff to increase survey awareness

____ 5.3 Explain roles and functions of regulatory agencies to staff

____ 5.4 Provide survey teams with requested documentation in accordance with agency policy

____ 5.5 Ensure that plans of correction are implemented

G. Agency Management Practices and Problems

1. Which of the following are the major problems in operating and maintaining this home? (mark all that apply)

   ___ a. Admissions policies
   ___ b. Community attitude toward residents
   ___ c. Certification and licensing
   ___ d. Developing individualized program plans
   ___ e. Difficulty finding qualified staff
   ___ f. Difficulty maintaining sufficient average daily resident population
   ___ g. Funding mechanism problems (e.g., late checks, county control)
   ___ h. Government regulations
   ___ i. Inadequate funds
   ___ j. Insurance problems
   ___ k. Lack of advocacy services
   ___ l. Lack of alternative community residential placements
   ___ m. Lack of community support services
   ___ n. Lack of coordination between provider agencies
   ___ o. Lack of follow-along services
   ___ p. Lack of program implementation
   ___ q. Lack of comprehensive state planning
   ___ r. Maintenance, physical plant, capital expenditures
   ___ s. Need for transportation services
   ___ t. Problems with residents
   ___ u. Problems with family members
   ___ v. Quality assurance
   ___ w. Relationships with board of directors
   ___ x. Staffing patterns and work conditions
   ___ y. Staff motivation
   ___ z. Staff training and development
   ___ aa. Staff turnover
   ___ bb. Start-up money and costs
   ___ cc. Unions/Labor relations
   ___ dd. Wage and hour considerations
   ___ ee. Workman's compensation
   ___ ff. Other _____

2. Which five of the following management practices are the most effective strategies your agency uses to address staffing issues for direct service staff members. (check five items from the list)

   ___ a. Communicate clear, understandable program objectives, and agency philosophy
   ___ b. Communicate the importance of each staff member to the agency
   ___ c. Encourage team work among staff
   ___ d. Encourage social involvement among employees
   ___ e. Establish effective communication among staff
   ___ f. Hire specific types of people/ask new hires for a time commitment.
   ___ g. Manage in a way that is perceived by staff to be fair
   ___ h. Provide a mechanism for complaints to management
   ___ i. Provide competitive pay and benefits
   ___ j. Provide employee fitness and wellness programs
   ___ k. Provide employee autonomy in their jobs, encourage creativity
   ___ l. Provide realistic information about the job to applicants.
   ___ m. Provide staff recognition
   ___ n. Support the staff members
   ___ o. Train supervisors to provide effective supervision to increase staff satisfaction with supervision
   ___ p. Treat staff fairly
   ___ q. Use a participatory management structure
   ___ r. Use a decentralized management structure - limit agency hierarchy
   ___ s. Use clear and understandable job roles and responsibilities
   ___ t. Other _____

H. Characteristics of the people living in this home. Please provide updated information about the people living in this home. The responses provided for last year's survey are enclosed for your reference.

Characteristic	1	2	3	4	5	6	7	8	9	10	11	12	13	14	15
Age (in years) 1 = 0-10 yrs, 2 = 11-20, 3 = 21-30, 4 = 31-40, 5 = 41-50, 6 = 51-60, 7 = 61-70, 8 = 71-80, 9 = 81-90															
Level of Mental Retardation 1 = normal (IQ 86+), 2 = borderline (IQ 71-85), 3 = mild (IQ 56-70), 4 = moderate (IQ 41-55), 5 = severe (IQ 26-40), 6 = profound (IQ 25 or less)															
Gender (0 = male, 1 = female)															
Year moved to this home 19___															
Moved here from a reg. treatment center (0 = no, 1 = yes)															
Autism (0 = no, 1 = yes)															
Blind or uncorrected vision impairment (0 = no, 1 = yes)															
Brain or neurological damage (0 = no, 1 = yes)															
Cerebral palsy (0 = no, 1 = yes)															
Deaf or uncorrected hearing impairment (0 = no, 1 = yes)															
Current epilepsy or seizure disorder (0 = no, 1 = yes)															
Mental illness - formal diagnosis (0 = no, 1 = yes)															
Specific planned intervention for challengingbehavior (e.g., aggression or self-injurious behavior) (0 = no, 1 = yes)															
Walks without assistance (0 = no, 1 = yes)															
Dresses without assistance (0 = no, 1 = yes)															
Eats without assistance (0 = no, 1 = yes)															
Independent in toileting (less than 1 day-time accident per month) (0 = no, 1 = yes)															
Communicates by talking (0 = no, 1 = yes)															

I. Open-Ended Questions

1. Describe any changes at this house or in your agency over the last 12 months that may have influenced recruitment, training or retention of direct service staff members.

_____

_____

_____

_____

_____

2. What do you believe are the most important factors influencing recruitment, training and retention of direct service staff members in this home?

_____

_____

_____

_____

_____

3. What 2 or 3 things could this agency do to help you do your job as a supervisor better?

_____

_____

_____

_____

_____

4. What (if any) positive or negative effect has participation in this study had on you and the direct service staff members working in this home?

_____

_____

_____

_____

_____

Thank you for your help.
Please return this survey to the University in the envelope provided.

Sherri Larson, ICI at U of MN
214B Pattee Hall, 150 Pillsbury Drive SE, Minneapolis, MN 55455
612-624-6024

FACILITY SURVEY (short version)

Date: _____   Facility ID: _____

Supervisor Name: _____ Facility Name: _____

Supervisor Title: _____ Agency ID: _____

Telephone Number: _____ Agency Name: _____

Instructions: This survey should be completed by the on-site supervisor responsible for hiring, firing, training and providing direct supervision to new direct service staff members in this home. Please answer each question as accurately as possible. If you do not understand a question, answer it as well as you can and write a note in the margin explaining your question. If there are questions that you cannot answer, please ask the person in your agency who has the answer or provide that person's name and phone number so we can contact them. *Your answers to these questions will be kept confidential and will not be shared with your employer.* If you have questions or need more information, please call Sherri Larson at 612-624-6024.

A. Supervisor Characteristics

1. How long have you worked in this home?**

   _____ years months

2. How many years of paid employment experience do you have working with people with developmental disabilities?

   _____ years

3. How many different program sites are you currently responsible for?

   _____ number of sites

4. How many hours per week (on average) do you spend working *at this home* in each of these roles? (Please provide a single number rather than a range of numbers.)

   _____ a. # of hrs working direct care

   _____ b. # of hours in supervisory or paperwork roles

5. Gender (mark one)

   _____ 0. male

   _____ 1. female

6. How old are you?

   _____ 1. 15-25 years

   _____ 2. 26-35 years

   _____ 3. 36-45 years

   _____ 4. 46-55 years

   _____ 5. 56-65 years

   _____ 6. 66-75 years

   _____ 7. 76-85 years

B. Facility characteristics

1. How many people with developmental disabilities live in this home?**

   _____ number of people

2. What year did *this home* begin providing residential services to persons with developmental disabilities?**

    19 _____

3. Which of these licensure categories best describes this home? (Mark one)**

    _____ 1. Intermediate Care Facility-Mental Retardation (ICF-MR, Rule 34)

    _____ 2. Supervised Living Services (SLS - Rule 42)

    _____ 3. Semi-independent Living Services (SILS - Rule 18)

    _____ 4. Other _____

4. What is the zip code for this home?

    _____

5. What city/municipality is this home located in (If in a metropolitan area, be specific - for example, if the home is in Bloomington, do not write Minneapolis)?**

    _____

6. What county is this home located in?**

    _____

7. What type of agency operates this home? (Mark one)**

    _____ 1. state (SOCS)

    _____ 2. county

    _____ 3. corporate profit

    _____ 4. corporate non-profit

    _____ 6. family (not incorporated)

8. What is the *total* dollar amount your agency receives *per day* to provide services to *all* of the people living in this home? (including room and board - if applicable)**

    $ _____ total per day

9. How many different residential sites does *your agency* operate in Minnesota?

    _____ # of different sites

10. What year did *your agency* begin providing services to persons with developmental disabilities?

    19 _____

C. **Characteristics of the Direct Service Staff Members:** Direct service staff members are people whose primary job responsibility is to provide support, training, supervision and personal assistance to people with developmental disabilities in this home.

1. On average, how many direct service staff members are on duty at the following times (including those who may be on break)?**

    Weekdays   Weekends

    _____ a. 7:30 am   _____ e. 7:30 am

    _____ b. 3:00 pm   _____ f. 3:00 pm

    _____ c. 7:30 pm   _____ g. 7:30 pm

    _____ d. 2:00 am   _____ h. 2:00 am

2. Please provide the following information about the *direct service staff members* currently working in this home.**

    _____ a. # direct service staff who work regular shifts in this home (counting all shifts, weekends, part-time and full-time; not including "on-call" staff)

    _____ b. # dss working regular shifts who are female

    _____ c. Total hours on schedule per pay period

    _____ d. # days in pay period

    _____ e. # unfilled or open positions

    _____ f. # of direct service staff who work *only* "on call" hours in this home

3. Please indicate the *current* beginning and maximum wage for direct service staff members now working in this home.**

Awake staff

a. $ _____/hr beginning wage (lowest)

b. $ _____ /hr current maximum wage

Sleep night staff

c. $ _____/hr beginning wage (lowest)

d. $ _____/hr current maximum wage

e. _____N/A sleep night staff not used

4. Do any paid direct service staff members live at this address? (mark one)**

_____ 0. no

_____ 1. yes

5. Are the direct service staff members in this home part of a union? (mark one)

_____ 0. no

_____ 1. yes

6. How many hours per week must a direct service employee work to be considered *full-time* by your agency?

_____ number of hours per week

7. How many hours per week must a *part-time* employee work to be eligible for paid leave time (e.g., sick, holiday or personal leave) from your agency?

_____ number of hours per week

8. How many hours per week must a *part-time* employee work to be eligible for benefits (e.g., health insurance) from your agency?

_____ number of hours per week

D. Recruitment and Retention Experiences

1. Do you have problems finding new direct service staff members? (mark one)**

_____ 0. no

_____ 1. yes

2. How useful are each of the following strategies in recruiting new direct service staff members to work in this home (rate each item)?

3 = Very helpful
2 = Somewhat helpful
1 = Not helpful
0 = Not used

_____ a. internal postings

_____ b. recruitment by current/former employees

_____ c. newspaper advertisements

_____ d. tv or radio advertisements

_____ e. employment/referral agency

_____ f. high school, technical college, or college placement office/job board

_____ g. other _____

3. *How many* new/returning/transferring direct service staff members *have been hired* to work regularly scheduled shifts at this house *during the last 12 months* (include persons who actually were paid for one or more hours of work. Do not include persons hired only to work temporary, on-call or fill-in hours).**

_____ number of different people

4. How satisfied were you that the last person you hired in a direct service staff position would fulfill the job requirements for that position? (mark one)

_____ 1. very satisfied

_____ 2. satisfied

_____ 3. somewhat satisfied

_____ 4. somewhat dissatisfied

_____ 5. dissatisfied

_____ 6. very dissatisfied

5. What are the primary limitations (if any) of recent applicants for direct service positions? (Mark all that apply)**

_____ a. None

_____ b. Lack of specific training

_____ c. Lack of basic communication skills (written, spoken)

_____ d. Lack of experience with people with developmental disabilities

_____ e. Lack of experience with job responsibilities

_____ f. Lack of maturity (e.g., experience managing a household, money management skills)

_____ g. other _____

6. Approximately how many applicants did you have the last time you hired a direct service staff member to work a weekend position in this home?

_____ number of applicants

7. The last time you hired a direct service staff member to work a weekend position, how many people did you extend a job offer to before the person who actually started working was hired (including the person who took the job)?

_____ # people offered the position

8. Counting all shifts (if applicable) and weekends, how many direct service staff members, including part-time persons (not including "on call" staff), left their direct service staff position for any reason during the last 12 months?**

_____ Total who left a direct service position in this home in the last 12 months

8a. For the direct service staff members who left in the last 12 months, how long had they worked in this home before leaving?

_____ a. # who had worked in this home less than 6 months

_____ b. # who had worked in this home 6 to 12 months

_____ c. # who had worked in this home over 12 months

9. How many direct service staff members from this home were promoted to supervisory or management positions in your agency in the last 12 months? (These supervisory or management positions may require some direct care.)

_____ number of people

10. How many direct service staff members from this home moved from part-time to full-time positions with this agency during the last 12 months?

_____ number of people

11. How much difficulty is caused by the amount of staff turnover in this home? (mark one)**

_____ 1. very much

_____ 2. much

_____ 3. little

_____ 4. very little or none

12. When do new direct service staff members first see a copy of their job description? (mark one)

_____ 1. when they get the application

_____ 2. when they return the application

_____ 3. after applying, before being hired

_____ 4. after being hired, before starting work

_____ 5. the first day of work

_____ 6. during the probationary period

_____ 7. after the probationary period

_____ 8. never

13. Do you use a temporary agency to provide direct service staff for this house?

_____ 0. no (skip to question 17)

_____ 1. yes

14. What company do you use?

_____

15. How many shifts did temporary agency staff work at this house in the last 30 days?

_____ number of shifts

16. How satisfied are you with the services of the temporary agency?

_____ 1. very satisfied

_____ 2. satisfied

_____ 3. dissatisfied

_____ 4. very dissatisfied

17. **Realistic job previews** tell applicants what to expect in a job, including features of the job that the person may not expect and may not like (e.g., having to work holidays, or working with individuals who may injure them). This information is presented before the applicant decides to take the job. Does your agency use realistic job previews when hiring direct service staff members? (mark one)

_____ 0. no (skip question 18)

_____ 1. yes

18. Which of the following strategies are used to provide information to applicants before a job is offered? (mark all that apply)

_____ a. none (we do not use RJP's)

_____ b. written information

_____ c. audio or video information

_____ d. verbal descriptions

_____ e. direct observation of people in the home

_____ f. other _____

19. Which five of the following management practices are the most effective strategies your agency uses to address staffing issues for direct service staff members. (check five items from the list)

_____ a. Communicate clear, understandable program objectives, and agency philosophy

_____ b. Communicate the importance of each staff member to the agency

_____ c. Encourage team work among staff

_____ d. Encourage social involvement among employees

_____ e. Establish effective communication among staff

_____ f. Hire specific types of people/ask new hires for a time commitment.

_____ g. Manage in a way that is perceived by staff to be fair

_____ h. Provide a mechanism for complaints to management

_____ i. Provide competitive pay and benefits

_____ j. Provide employee fitness and wellness programs

_____ k. Provide employee autonomy in their jobs, encourage creativity

_____ l. Provide realistic information about the job to applicants.

_____ m. Provide staff recognition

_____ n. Support the staff members

_____ o. Train supervisors to provide effective supervision to increase staff satisfaction with supervision

_____ p. Treat staff fairly

_____ q. Use a participatory management structure

_____ r. Use a decentralized management structure - limit agency hierarchy

_____ s. Use clear and understandable job roles and responsibilities

_____ t. Other _____

E. Characteristics of the People Living in This Home

1. _____ Number of people with developmental disabilities who live in this home?

2. How many are in each age range?

   _____ a. 0-10 years,

   _____ b. 11-20 years,

   _____ c. 21-30 years,

   _____ d. 31-40 years,

   _____ e. 41-50 years,

   _____ f. 51-60 years,

   _____ g. 61-70 years,

   _____ h. 71-80 years,

   _____ i. 81-90 years

3. How many have each level of mental retardation?

   _____ a. normal (IQ 86+)

   _____ b. borderline (IQ 71-85)

   _____ c. mild (IQ 56-70)

   _____ d. moderate (IQ 41-55)

   _____ e. severe (IQ 26-40)

   _____ f. profound (IQ 25 or less)

4. _____ Number of residents who are female.

5. _____ Number of residents who moved here from a regional treatment center.

6. _____ Number of residents who are blind or have uncorrected vision impairments.

7. _____ Number of residents who are deaf or have uncorrected hearing impairments.

8. _____ Number of residents who have a specific planned intervention for challenging behavior (e.g., aggression or self-injurious behavior).

9. _____ Number of residents who walk without assistance.

10. _____ Number of residents who are independent in toileting (less than 1 day-time accident per month).

11. _____ Number of residents who communicate by talking.

F. Open-Ended Questions

1. Describe any changes at this house or in your agency over the last 12 months that may have influenced recruitment, training or retention of direct service staff members.

_____

_____

_____

_____

_____

2. What do you believe are the most important factors influencing recruitment, training and retention of direct service staff members in this home?

_____

_____

_____

_____

_____

3. What 2 or 3 things could this agency do to help you do your job as a supervisor better?

_____

_____

_____

_____

_____

4. What (if any) positive or negative effect has participation in this study had on you and the direct service staff members working in this home?

_____

_____

_____

_____

_____

Thank you for your help.
Please return this survey to the University in the envelope provided.

Sherri Larson, ICI at U of MN
214B Pattee Hall, 150 Pillsbury Drive SE, Minneapolis, MN 55455
612-624-6024

APPENDIX B
STAFF SURVEYS

STAFF SURVEY (Time 1—First day of work)

Date: _____

Staff Name: _____

Staff Title: _____

Telephone Number: _____

Staff ID: _____

Facility Name: _____

Facility ID: _____

Agency ID: _____

Instructions: This survey should be filled out <u>before</u> you begin your direct service staff responsibilities. Please answer each question as accurately as possible. If you do not understand a question, answer it as well as you can and note your question(s) in the margin. <u>Your answers to these questions will be kept confidential and will not be shared with your employer.</u> When you have completed this survey please return it to the University in the envelope provided. If you have questions, you can contact Sherri Larson at 612-624-6024. Thank you.

A. Background information

1. Gender (mark one)

   _____ 0.   male

   _____ 1.   female

2. What is your birth date?

   _____ month   _____ year

3. How would you describe your ethnic background? (mark one)

   _____ 1.   White

   _____ 2.   Black

   _____ 3.   Hispanic

   _____ 4.   Asian, Pacific Islander

   _____ 5.   American Indian, Alaskan Native

   _____ 6.   other _____

4. What is your marital status? (mark one)

   _____ 0.   not married

   _____ 1.   married

5. Are you a primary source of financial support for any legal dependents such as children or elderly parents? (mark one)

   _____ 0.   no

   _____ 1.   yes

B. Education and Experience

1. How many years of paid employment experience do you have working with people with developmental disabilities?

   _____ years _____ months

2. What was your official starting date in this home?

   _____ month   _____ year

3. How long have you worked for this agency?

   _____ years _____ months

4. How did you hear about this job (mark the <u>most important</u> source)?

_____ 1. I worked for this agency before

_____ 2. A current/former employee of this agency

_____ 3. A friend who works for another agency serving people with developmental disabilities

_____ 4. A person with developmental disabilities or their family

_____ 5. Media advertisement (TV, radio, newspaper)

_____ 6. Employment/referral agency

_____ 7. High school or college placement office

_____ 8. Explored the possibility on my own initiative

_____ 9. Other _____

5. How many years of school have you finished? (circle one)

9 (Junior High School)

10

11

12 (High school graduate or GED)

13

14 (Associate or 2 year degree)

15

16 (Four year degree)

17

18 (Master's level degree)

19

20

21 (Doctoral degree)

6. Did you take any courses on mental retardation or on working with people who have disabilities as part of your general education (e.g., in college or technical school)? (mark one)

_____ 0. no

_____ 1. yes

7. Are you currently enrolled in vocational/technical school or college? (mark one)

_____ 0. no

_____ 1. yes

7a. If yes, do you intend to continue working in your present position when you have completed your education? (mark one)

_____ 0. no

_____ 1. yes

8. How much did you know about the following before you accepted this job? (circle one number for each item)

a. This agency's reputation

1 2 3 4 5
Nothing   A great deal

b. Your pay and benefits

1 2 3 4 5
Nothing   A great deal

c. The working conditions in this home

1 2 3 4 5
Nothing   A great deal

d. The types of tasks you would be doing

1 2 3 4 5
Nothing   A great deal

e. What the other direct care staff would be like

1 2 3 4 5
Nothing   A great deal

f. What your supervisor would be like

1 2 3 4 5
Nothing   A great deal

g. Needs and characteristics of the residents in this home

1 2 3 4 5
Nothing   A great deal

9. How many job offers (including this one) have you had in the last month?

_____ number of offers

10. Of the following factors, which was the most important influence on your decision to take this job. (Mark one)

_____ 1. I needed the income or benefits provided by this job.

_____ 2. The job provided training or experience working with people with developmental disabilities that I need to meet my career goals.

_____ 3. I have a special interest in working with the people in this home/people with developmental disabilities.

_____ 4. Other _____

C. Job Characteristics

1. How many hours will you work per week in this home?

_____ hours

2. During which time period will most of your working hours fall? (mark one)

_____ 1. 7:00 AM to 3:00 PM

_____ 2. 3:00 PM to 11:00 PM

_____ 3. 11:00 PM to 7:00 AM - awake

_____ 4. 11:00 PM to 7:00 AM - asleep

3. Is this group home/program site your primary residence? (mark one) (i.e., Do you live here?)

_____ 0. no

_____ 1. yes

4. What is your current salary?

$ _____ per hour

5. How many weekend days will you work per month? (A shift that lasts more than 8 hours and occurs on both Saturday and Sunday should be counted as 2 days for this question).

_____ days per month

6. How much pay do you want compared to what you currently get at this job? (mark one)

I want:

_____ 1. much more pay

_____ 2. somewhat more pay

_____ 3. no more or no less pay

_____ 4. somewhat less pay

_____ 5. much less pay

7. How much difference is there between the hourly pay you get for this job and the hourly pay you got for your previous job? (mark one)

This job provides:

_____ 1. much more pay

_____ 2. somewhat more pay

_____ 3. no more or no less pay

_____ 4. somewhat less pay

_____ 5. much less pay

_____ 6. this is my first job

8. How much difference is there between the hourly pay you get for this job and the hourly pay you need to meet your basic expenses? (mark one)

I need:

_____ 1. much more pay

_____ 2. somewhat more pay

_____ 3. no more or no less pay

_____ 4. somewhat less pay

_____ 5. much less pay

D. Job Expectations

1. For each item on this chart indicate whether you think each job characteristic will be present in your job. Then indicate how important this job characteristic is to you.

Job Characteristic		I **expect** this job feature to occur in this job 1 = Strongly agree 2 = Agree 3 = Neither agree or disagree 4 = Disagree 5 = Strongly disagree	This characteristic is **important** to me 1 = Strongly agree 2 = Agree 3 = Neither agree or disagree 4 = Disagree 5 = Strongly disagree
a.	I will be able to keep busy all the time	1 2 3 4 5	1 2 3 4 5
b.	I will be able to work independently	1 2 3 4 5	1 2 3 4 5
c.	I will be able to do different things from time to time	1 2 3 4 5	1 2 3 4 5
d.	I will be respected by the community	1 2 3 4 5	1 2 3 4 5
e.	I will have a good boss	1 2 3 4 5	1 2 3 4 5
f.	My supervisor will be competent in making decisions	1 2 3 4 5	1 2 3 4 5
g.	I will be doing things that don't go against my conscience	1 2 3 4 5	1 2 3 4 5
h.	My job will provide steady employment	1 2 3 4 5	1 2 3 4 5
i.	I will have a chance to do things for other people	1 2 3 4 5	1 2 3 4 5
j.	I will have a chance to tell other people what to do	1 2 3 4 5	1 2 3 4 5
k.	I will be doing things that use my abilities	1 2 3 4 5	1 2 3 4 5
l.	I will like the way company policies are put into practice	1 2 3 4 5	1 2 3 4 5
m.	I will be satisfied with my pay and the amount of work I do	1 2 3 4 5	1 2 3 4 5
n.	I will have chances for advancement on this job	1 2 3 4 5	1 2 3 4 5

o.	I will have freedom to use my own judgement	1	2	3	4	5	1	2	3	4	5
p.	I will be able to try my own methods of doing the job	1	2	3	4	5	1	2	3	4	5
q.	I will be satisfied with the working conditions	1	2	3	4	5	1	2	3	4	5
r.	My co-workers will get along together	1	2	3	4	5	1	2	3	4	5
s.	I will get praise for doing a good job	1	2	3	4	5	1	2	3	4	5
t.	I will get a feeling of accomplishment from the job	1	2	3	4	5	1	2	3	4	5
u.	Adequate equipment and supplies will be available	1	2	3	4	5	1	2	3	4	5
v.	Adequate money and transportation will be available for community activities	1	2	3	4	5	1	2	3	4	5
w.	My fellow workers will provide advice and support	1	2	3	4	5	1	2	3	4	5
x.	My supervisor will provide advice and support	1	2	3	4	5	1	2	3	4	5
y.	Backup support will be available for emergencies	1	2	3	4	5	1	2	3	4	5
z.	Training and technical assistance will be available	1	2	3	4	5	1	2	3	4	5

E. Employment Outlook

1. How do you rate your chances of still working in this home: (Circle one response for each item.)

7 = Excellent   3 = Not so Good
6 = Very Good   2 = Bad
5 = Good   1 = Terrible
4 = So-So

a. Three months from now

7   6   5   4   3   2   1
Excellent   Terrible

b. Six months from now

7   6   5   4   3   2   1
Excellent   Terrible

c. One year from now

7   6   5   4   3   2   1
Excellent   Terrible

d. Two years from now

7   6   5   4   3   2   1
Excellent   Terrible

2. Given your age, education, and the general economic condition, what do you feel your chance is of attaining a suitable position in some other organization? (mark one)

_____ 1. Excellent
_____ 2. Very Good
_____ 3. Good
_____ 4. So-So
_____ 5. Not So Good
_____ 6. Bad
_____ 7. Terrible

3. How many years do you plan to continue to work in your current position in this home? (make your best estimate if you are not sure).

_____ years

4. Which of the following job search activities have you done during the last 30 days? (mark all that apply)

_____ a. reading help wanted ads
_____ b. talked with friends and business acquaintances to identify possible job openings
_____ c. contacting an employment agency
_____ d. calling agencies to find out if they have any job openings
_____ e. gathering information about specific agencies (for example, from the library)

_____ f. interviews with agencies to find out about the agency (not a job interview)
_____ g. submitting job applications to agencies without a specific opening
_____ h. submitting job applications for a specific opening
_____ i. job interview for a specific opening
_____ j. other

5. How do you rate your chances of: (Circle one response for each item.)

7 = Excellent   3 = Not so Good
6 = Very Good   2 = Bad
5 = Good   1 = Terrible
4 = So-So

a. Quitting this job in the next three months

    7   6   5   4   3   2   1
    Excellent   Terrible

b. Quitting this job sometime in the next six months

    7   6   5   4   3   2   1
    Excellent   Terrible

c. Quitting this job sometime in the next year

    7   6   5   4   3   2   1
    Excellent   Terrible

d. Quitting this job sometime in the next two years

    7   6   5   4   3   2   1
    Excellent   Terrible

STAFF SURVEY
(Time 2, 3, 4—After 30 days, 6 months, 12 months)

Date: _____   Staff ID: _____

Staff Name: _____   Facility Name: _____

Staff Title: _____   Facility ID: _____

Telephone Number: _____   Agency ID: _____

Instructions: This survey should be filled out after you have been on the job for one month. Please answer each question as accurately as possible. If you do not understand a question, answer it as well as you can and note your question(s) in the margin. Your answers to these questions will be kept confidential and will not be shared with your employer.

Also complete the blue Leader Behavior Descriptive Questionnaire focusing on your thoughts about your supervisor in this home. When you have completed both forms, please return them to the University in the envelope provided. If you have questions, you can contact Sherri Larson at 612-624-6024. Thank you.

A. General Information

1. How many different positions have you had in this home since you were hired? (If you are still in the same position you were first hired for write 1 on the blank)

   _____ number of different positions

2. How many hours do you work per week in this home?

   _____ number of hours per week

3. During which time period do most of your working hours fall? (mark one)

   _____ 1. 7:00 AM to 3:00 PM

   _____ 2. 3:00 PM to 11:00 PM

   _____ 3. 11:00 PM to 7:00 AM - awake

   _____ 4. 11:00 PM to 7:00 AM - asleep

4. Is this group home/program site your primary residence (i.e., Do you live here)? (mark one)

   _____ 0. no

   _____ 1. yes

5. What is your current salary?

   $ _____ per hour

6. How many weekend days do you work per month? (A shift that lasts more than 8 hours and occurs on both Saturday and Sunday should be counted as 2 days for this question).

   _____ number of weekend days per month

7. When did you first see a copy of your job description? (mark one)

_____ 1. when I got the application		_____ 5. the first day of work
_____ 2. when I returned the application		_____ 6. during the probationary period
_____ 3. after applying, before being hired		_____ 7. after the probationary period
_____ 4. after being hired, before starting work		_____ 8. never

B. Organizational Commitment

Listed below are a series of statements that represent possible feelings that individuals might have about the company or organization for which they work. With respect to your own feelings about the particular organization for which you are now working, please indicate the degree of your agreement or disagreement with each statement by circling one of the seven alternatives.

1	2	3	4	5	6	7
Strongly Disagree	Moderately Disagree	Slightly Disagree	Neither Agree or Disagree	Slightly Agree	Moderately Agree	Strongly Disagree

		SD						SA
1.	I am willing to put in a great deal of effort beyond what is normally expected in order to help this organization be successful.	1	2	3	4	5	6	7
2.	I talk up this organization to my friends as a great organization to work for.	1	2	3	4	5	6	7
3.	I feel very little loyalty to this organization.	1	2	3	4	5	6	7
4.	I would accept almost any type of job assignment in order to keep working for this organization.	1	2	3	4	5	6	7
5.	I find that my values and the organization's values are similar.	1	2	3	4	5	6	7
6.	I am proud to tell others that I am part of this organization.	1	2	3	4	5	6	7
7.	I could just as well be working for a different organization as long as the type of work was similar.	1	2	3	4	5	6	7
8.	This organization really inspires the very best in me in the way of job performance.	1	2	3	4	5	6	7
9.	It would take very little change in my present circumstances to cause me to leave this organization.	1	2	3	4	5	6	7

10.	I am extremely glad that I chose this organization to work for over others I was considering at the time I joined.	1	2	3	4	5	6	7
11.	There's not too much to be gained by sticking with this organization indefinitely.	1	2	3	4	5	6	7
12.	Often, I find it difficult to agree with this organization's policies on important matters relating to its employees.	1	2	3	4	5	6	7
13.	I really care about the fate of this organization.	1	2	3	4	5	6	7
14.	For me this is the best of all possible organizations for which to work	1	2	3	4	5	6	7
15.	Deciding to work for this organization was a definite mistake on my part.	1	2	3	4	5	6	7

C. Opinions About Your Work Role

1. Are you treated as an important and equal member of the interdisciplinary team? (multi-agency group that makes decisions about individual residents' programs and plans) (mark one)

    _____ 1. definitely yes

    _____ 2. somewhat yes

    _____ 3. neither yes or no

    _____ 4. somewhat no

    _____ 5. definitely no

2. Do you receive the support you need from case managers and staff from other programs to be as effective as you would like with the residents? (mark one)

    _____ 1. definitely yes

    _____ 2. somewhat yes

    _____ 3. neither yes or no

    _____ 4. somewhat no

    _____ 5. definitely no

3. Have your job responsibilities and working conditions turned out to be what you expected when you took this job? (mark one)

    _____ 1. definitely yes

    _____ 2. somewhat yes

    _____ 3. neither yes or no

    _____ 4. somewhat no

    _____ 5. definitely no

4. Overall, does this job meet your original expectations? (mark one)

    _____ 1. definitely yes

    _____ 2. somewhat yes

    _____ 3. neither yes or no

    _____ 4. somewhat no

    _____ 5. definitely no

D. Job Satisfaction (Minnesota Satisfaction Questionnaire)

The Minnesota Satisfaction Questionnaire could not be included here because it is a copyrighted instrument.

E. Satisfaction with supports and resources

	Very Dissatisfied 1	Dissatisfied 2	Neutral 3	Satisfied 4	Very Satisfied 5		

On my present job, this is how I feel about...	VD				VS
21. Availability of needed equipment and supplies	1	2	3	4	5
22. Availability of money and transportation for community activities	1	2	3	4	5
23. Availability of advice and support from fellow workers	1	2	3	4	5
24. Availability of advice and support from my supervisor	1	2	3	4	5
25. Availability of backup support to handle emergencies	1	2	3	4	5
26. Availability of training and technical assistance	1	2	3	4	5

F. Training Experiences

Please answer these questions about the training you have received from the agency in which you now work. Circle the number based on this scale that most accurately reflects your opinion.

	Strongly Disagree 1	Disagree 2	Undecided 3	Agree 4	Strongly Agree 5

The orientation and training I have received so far has:	SD				SA
1. Prepared me to complete most of my specific job responsibilities.	1	2	3	4	5
2. Assisted me to develop my resident interaction skills.	1	2	3	4	5
3. Helped me to improve resident quality of life.	1	2	3	4	5
4. Missed important information I need to perform my job.	1	2	3	4	5
5. Been worthwhile.	1	2	3	4	5
6. Not sparked my interest.	1	2	3	4	5

7. I would recommend the orientation and training I have received so far to all new employees of this agency. (mark one)

_____ 1. Strongly disagree

_____ 2. Disagree

_____ 3. Undecided

_____ 4. Agree

_____ 5. Strongly agree

8. This agency should develop a new orientation and training program. (mark one)

_____ 1. Strongly disagree

_____ 2. Disagree

_____ 3. Undecided

_____ 4. Agree

_____ 5. Strongly agree

G. Supervisor Characteristics

1. Does your supervisor make good decisions about daily work schedules? (mark one)

_____ 1. always

_____ 2. often

_____ 3. occasionally

_____ 4. seldom

_____ 5. never

2. Does your supervisor make good decisions about resident training and programs? (mark one)

_____ 1. always

_____ 2. often

_____ 3. occasionally

_____ 4. seldom

_____ 5. never

3. Does your supervisor look out for the personal welfare of residents? (mark one)

_____ 1. always

_____ 2. often

_____ 3. occasionally

_____ 4. seldom

_____ 5. never

H. Employment Outlook

1. How do you rate your chances of still working in this home: (Circle one response for each item.)

7 = Excellent   3 = Not so Good
6 = Very Good   2 = Bad
5 = Good   1 = Terrible
4 = So-So

a. Three months from now

7   6   5   4   3   2   1
Excellent   Terrible

b. Six months from now

7   6   5   4   3   2   1
Excellent   Terrible

c. One year from now

7   6   5   4   3   2   1
Excellent   Terrible

d. Two years from now

7   6   5   4   3   2   1
Excellent   Terrible

2. Given your age, education, and the general economic condition, what do you feel your chance is of attaining a suitable position in some other organization? (mark one)

_____ 1. Excellent

_____ 2. Very Good

_____ 3. Good

_____ 4. So-So

_____ 5. Not So Good

_____ 6. Bad

_____ 7. Terrible

3. If you had left this job during the past month, would your next job probably have been better or worse than the job you have now? (mark one)

_____ 1. Definitely worse
_____ 2. Probably worse
_____ 3. Probably the same
_____ 4. Probably better
_____ 5. Definitely better

4. During the past month, how hard would it have been for you to find a job with another employer with approximately the same income and benefits you have now? (mark one)

_____ 1. Not at all difficult
_____ 2. Not very difficult
_____ 3. Moderately difficult
_____ 4. Very difficult
_____ 5. Extremely difficult

5. As of the past month, how confident were you that you would find a satisfactory job if you had quit this one? (mark one)

_____ 1. Extremely confident
_____ 2. Very confident
_____ 3. Moderately confident
_____ 4. Not very confident
_____ 5. Not at all confident

6. All things considered, as of the past month how did other job opportunities compare to your current job? (mark one)

_____ 1. Other jobs were much worse
_____ 2. Other jobs were somewhat worse
_____ 3. Other jobs were about the same
_____ 4. Other jobs were somewhat better
_____ 5. Other jobs were much better

7. How likely is it that you might be fired or laid off? (mark one)

_____ 1. highly unlikely
_____ 2. unlikely
_____ 3. somewhat unlikely
_____ 4. neither likely or unlikely
_____ 5. somewhat likely
_____ 6. likely
_____ 7. highly likely

8. How many years do you plan to continue to work in your current position in this home? (please make your best estimate even if you are not sure).

_____ years

9. How likely is it that you will be promoted by this company within the next 2 years?

_____ 1. very likely
_____ 2. somewhat likely
_____ 3. so-so
_____ 4. somewhat unlikely
_____ 5. very unlikely

10. How important is it to you that this company provide promotion opportunities to direct service staff?

_____ 1. very important
_____ 2. important
_____ 3. so-so
_____ 4. somewhat unimportant
_____ 5. not important at all

11. Which of the following job search activities have you done during the last 30 days? (mark all that apply)

_____ a. reading help wanted ads
_____ b. talked with friends and business acquaintances to identify possible job openings

_____ c.	contacting an employment agency

_____ d.	calling agencies to find out if they have any job openings

_____ e.	gathering information about specific agencies (for example, from the library)

_____ f.	interviews to find out about an agency (not a job interview)

_____ g.	submitting job applications to agencies without a specific opening

_____ h.	submitting job applications for a specific opening

_____ i.	job interview for a specific opening

_____ j.	other

_____ k.	none of the above

12. How do you rate your chances of: (Circle one response for each item.)

7 = Excellent   3 = Not so Good
6 = Very Good   2 = Bad
5 = Good   1 = Terrible
4 = So-So

a.	Quitting this job in the next three months

    7   6   5   4   3   2   1
    Excellent   Terrible

b.	Quitting this job sometime in the next six months

    7   6   5   4   3   2   1
    Excellent   Terrible

c.	Quitting this job sometime in the next year

    7   6   5   4   3   2   1
    Excellent   Terrible

d.	Quitting this job sometime in the next two years

    7   6   5   4   3   2   1
    Excellent   Terrible

13. Give an example of one or two specific incidents that made you decide you want to stay on this job.

_____

_____

14. Give an example of one or two specific incidents that made you decide you want to leave this job.

_____

_____

15. What could your employer do to make your job better?

_____

_____

16. What was the hardest part of your first month on this job?

_____

_____

17. List the four topics on which you most need training right now:

a. _____
b. _____
c. _____
d. _____

I. Advice to New Employees

1. If your best friend was considering a job like yours at this home, what 2 or 3 things would you tell him or her before he or she decided whether or not to take the job? Give specific examples.

a. _____
b. _____
c. _____

STAFF SURVEY
(Time 2a—After 30 days—continued)

Date: _____   Facility Name: _____

Staff Name: _____   Facility ID: _____

Staff ID: _____   Agency ID: _____

Organizational Socialization

Instructions: Listed below are a series of statements about the experiences you had as you began your job in this home. Please indicate the degree of your agreement or disagreement with each statement by circling one of the seven possible answers.

1	2	3	4	5	6	7
Strongly Disagree	Moderately Disagree	Slightly Disagree	Neither Agree or Disagree	Slightly Agree	Moderately Agree	Strongly Disagree

SD   SA

A. In my first several weeks on the job, I have been extensively involved with other new staff in common training activities.   1   2   3   4   5   6   7

B. Other new staff have been instrumental in helping me to understand my job requirements.   1   2   3   4   5   6   7

C. This organization puts all newcomers through the same set of learning experiences.   1   2   3   4   5   6   7

D. Most of my training has been carried out apart from other newcomers.   1   2   3   4   5   6   7

E. There is a sense of "being in the same boat" or in similar situations amongst newcomers in this agency.   1   2   3   4   5   6   7

2A. I have been through a set of training experiences which are specifically designed to give newcomers a thorough knowledge of job related skills.   1   2   3   4   5   6   7

2B. During my training for this job, I was normally physically apart from non-newcomers in the organization.   1   2   3   4   5   6   7

2C. I did not perform any of my normal job responsibilities until I was thoroughly familiar with the procedures and work methods of the job site.   1   2   3   4   5   6   7

		SD						SA
2D.	Much of my job knowledge has been acquired informally on a trial and error basis.	1	2	3	4	5	6	7
2E.	I have been very aware that I am seen as "learning the ropes" in this job.	1	2	3	4	5	6	7
3A.	There is a clear pattern in the way one job assignment leads to another in this agency.	1	2	3	4	5	6	7
3B.	Each state of the training process builds upon the job knowledge gained during the preceding stages of the process.	1	2	3	4	5	6	7
3C.	Movement of staff from job assignment to job assignment to build up experience and a track record is very apparent in this agency.	1	2	3	4	5	6	7
3D.	This agency does not put newcomers through an identifiable sequence of learning experiences.	1	2	3	4	5	6	7
3E.	The steps in the career ladder are clearly specified in this agency.	1	2	3	4	5	6	7
4A.	I can predict my future career path in this agency observing other people's experiences.	1	2	3	4	5	6	7
4B.	I have good knowledge of the time it will take me to go through the various stages of the training process in this agency.	1	2	3	4	5	6	7
4C.	The way in which my progress through this organization will follow a fixed timetable of events has been clearly communicated to me.	1	2	3	4	5	6	7
4D.	I have little idea when to expect a new training session or job assignment in this agency.	1	2	3	4	5	6	7
4E.	Most of my knowledge of what may happen to me in the future comes informally, through the grapevine, rather than through regular agency channels.	1	2	3	4	5	6	7
5A.	Experienced agency members see advising or training newcomers as one of their main job responsibilities in this agency.	1	2	3	4	5	6	7
5B.	I am gaining a clear understanding of my role in this organization by observing my senior coworkers.	1	2	3	4	5	6	7
5C.	I have not received guidance from experienced staff as to how I should perform my job.	1	2	3	4	5	6	7

	SD						SA
5D. I have little or no access to people who have previously performed my role.	1	2	3	4	5	6	7
5E. I have been generally left alone to discover what my role should be in this agency.	1	2	3	4	5	6	7
6A. I have been made to feel that my skills and abilities are very important in this agency.	1	2	3	4	5	6	7
6B. Almost all of my coworkers have been supportive of me personally.	1	2	3	4	5	6	7
6C. I have had to change my attitudes and values to be accepted in this agency.	1	2	3	4	5	6	7
6D. My coworkers have gone out of their way to help me adjust to this job.	1	2	3	4	5	6	7
6E. I feel that experienced staff have held me at a distance until I conform to their expectations.	1	2	3	4	5	6	7

Please return this survey, your Time 2 survey, and the Leader Behavior Description Questionnaire in the envelope provided.

If you have questions, please contact
Sherri Larson at 612-624-6024. Thank you.

STAFF SURVEY
(Time 5—After giving notice)

ate: _____   Staff ID: _____

taff Name: _____   Facility Name: _____

taff Title: _____   Facility ID: _____

elepnone Number: _____   Agency ID: _____

nstructions: This survey will gather information about direct service staff members who re leaving their positions. Please answer each question as accurately as possible. If you do ot understand a question, answer it as well as you can and note your question(s) in the argin. Your answers to these questions will be kept confidential and will not be shared ith your employer. When you have completed this survey, please return it to the University in the envelope provided. If you have questions, you can contact Sherri Larson at 612-24-6024. Thank you.

. What is your official last date of employ-ment in the position?

_____ month _____ day _____ year

2. How many different positions have you had <u>in this home</u> since you were hired? (If you are still in the same position you were first hired for write 1 on the blank)

_____ number of positions

or the next set of questions use this scale:

Strongly Agree 1	Agree 2	Undecided 3	Disagree 4	Strongly Disagree 5

	SA				SD
3. It was entirely my decision to leave the organization.	1	2	3	4	5
4. It was at least partly the organization's decision that I leave.	1	2	3	4	5
5. Informally, I was encouraged to leave the organization.	1	2	3	4	5
6. I am certain that the organization wanted me to stay.	1	2	3	4	5
7. The decision was made mostly by the organization.	1	2	3	4	5
8. The organization no longer needed me.	1	2	3	4	5
9. The decision to leave was mostly mine.	1	2	3	4	5

	SA				SD
10. The decision to leave could not have been avoided by the organization.	1	2	3	4	5
11. The organization could have made changes which would have led me to stay.	1	2	3	4	5
12. The reasons I left have nothing to do with the organization.	1	2	3	4	5
13. The organization could have convinced me to stay.	1	2	3	4	5
14. The factors influencing the decision to leave were beyond the organization's control.	1	2	3	4	5
15. I would have stayed if things were better at the organization.	1	2	3	4	5
16. The reasons I left do not concern my career at the organization.	1	2	3	4	5

17. What were the primary reasons for your decision to leave your position?

_____

_____

_____

18. Describe the type of position (if any) you plan to take after you leave this position (e.g., supervisor in a group home, job coach at a DAC, teller at a bank).

_____

_____

19. If your best friend was considering a job like yours at this home, what 2 or 3 things would you tell him or her before he or she decided whether or not to take the job? Give specific examples.

a. _____

_____

b. _____

_____

c. _____

_____

20. Give examples of one or two specific incidents that made you decide to leave this job.

_____

_____

_____

_____

.. What, if anything, could this agency have done to make you stay in this position?

_____

_____

_____

Thank you for your help. Please return this survey
to the University in the envelope provided.

ICI at U of MN, 214B Pattee Hall, 150 Pillsbury Dr. SE.,
Mpls, MN 55455 (612) 624-6024

SUPERVISOR EXIT QUESTIONNAIRE

Facility Name: _____

Facility ID: _____

Direct Services Staff Name: _____

Direct Services Staff ID: _____

Supervisor Name: _____

Supervisor ID: _____

Instructions: Please answer these questions about the direct service staff member who left.

What is the employees' official last date of employment in the position?

_____ month _____ day _____ year

Was this employee terminated involuntarily? (mark one)

_____ 1. no

_____ 2. yes

Would you rehire the employee who left? (mark one)

_____ 1. Under no circumstances

_____ 2. Unlikely

_____ 3. Uncertain

_____ 4. Possibly

_____ 5. Definitely

How would you rate the job performance of the employee who left? (mark one)

_____ 1. Inadequate

_____ 2. Barely adequate

_____ 3. Adequate

_____ 4. Good

_____ 5. Excellent

Use the following scale for the next set of questions:

1 Strongly Agree
2 Agree
3 Neither Agree or Disagree
4 Disagree
5 Strongly Disagree

_____ 5. It was entirely the employee's decision to leave the organization.

_____ 6. It was at least partly the organization's decision that he/she leave.

_____ 7. Informally, he/she was encouraged to leave the organization.

_____ 8. I am certain that the organization wanted the employee to stay.

_____ 9. The decision was made mostly by the organization.

_____ 10. The organization no longer needed the employee.

_____ 11. The decision to leave was mostly the employee's.

_____ 12. The decision to leave could not have been avoided by the organization.

_____ 13. The organization could have made changes which would have led the employee to stay.

_____ 14. The reasons the employee left have nothing to do with the organization.

_____ 15. The organization could have convinced the employee to stay.

_____ 16. The factors influencing the decision to leave were beyond the organization's control.

_____ 17. The employee would have stayed if things were better at the organization.

_____ 18. The reasons the employee left do not concern his/her career at the organization.

19. In general, how easy would it be to find someone who would do as good a job as the employee who left? (mark one)

_____ 1. very easy

_____ 2. easy

_____ 3. neither easy or difficult

_____ 4. difficult

_____ 5. very difficult

20. Where did the staff member who left go.

_____ 1. Same agency - promotion

_____ 2. Same agency - lateral move

_____ 3. Left agency

21. Will the staff member who left continue to work "on-call" hours at this site?

_____ 0. no

_____ 1. yes